£29.50

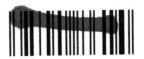

# Ostomy Care and the Cancer Patient

## Surgical and Clinical Considerations

# Ostomy Care and the Cancer Patient
## Surgical and Clinical Considerations

Edited by

## Dorothy B. Smith, R.N., M.S., E.T.
### Department of Nursing

## Douglas E. Johnson, M.D.
### Ashbel Smith Professor of Urology

The University of Texas M. D. Anderson Hospital
and Tumor Institute at Houston
Houston, Texas

Grune & Stratton, Inc.
Harcourt Brace Jovanovich, Publishers
Orlando    New York    San Diego    Boston    London
San Francisco    Tokyo    Sydney    Toronto

**Library of Congress Cataloging-in-Publication Data**

Ostomy care and the cancer patient.

Includes index.
1. Enterostomy. 2. Enterostomy—Complications and
sequelae. 3. Ostomates—Care and treatment.
4. Ostomates—Psychology. 5. Cancer—Surgery—
Patients—Rehabilitation. I. Smith, Dorothy B.
II. Johnson, Douglas E., 1934- . [DNLM:
1. Gastroenterostomy—nursing. 2. Neoplasms—nursing.
3. Neoplasms—surgery. 4. Urinary Diversions—nursing.
WY 156 085]
RD540.087 1986                617'.554                86-4684
ISBN 0-8089-1807-0

Grune & Stratton, Inc.
Orlando, Florida 32887

Distributed in the United Kingdom by
Grune & Stratton, Ltd.
24/28 Oval Road, London NW 1

Library of Congress Catalog Number 86-4684
International Standard Book Number 0-8089-1807-9
Printed in the United States of America

86  87  88  89     10  9  8  7  6  5  4  3  2  1

# Contents

# Preface

This year more than 100,000 men, women, and children in the United States will undergo ostomy surgery. In the majority of instances their surgery will be required either as primary treatment of a malignant disease or as management of complications stemming from a malignancy. Although major advances in cancer treatments have occurred during the last several decades, the emphasis on rehabilitating a person with an ostomy has not kept pace with our other achievements.

We tend to forget that creating an ostomy for a patient with cancer is not a new procedure. In 1826, Lisfranc excised a rectal carcinoma and constructed a perineal colostomy. A few years later, in Paris, Amussat developed the lumbar colostomy. Few major changes have been made in the principles of colostomy construction since 1884, when Maydl suggested the use of a goose quill bridge to support a loop colostomy on the abdominal wall. Similarly, before the turn of the century cystectomy and urinary diversion were being combined to treat bladder cancer. However, radical exenterative surgery requiring either a fecal or a urinary ostomy was performed infrequently until the late 1940s, when the pioneering work of Brunschwig, Bricker, and Appleby demonstrated improved survival rates for patients operated on for rectal and gynecologic malignancies. Since then, the amounts of exenterative surgery and the number of accompanying ostomies have increased rapidly.

Early ostomies were managed by absorbent waddings held in place by a belt during the day and a binder or closely fitting wrapper at night. Frequently, for support, the patient wore a round piece of cardboard or celluloid the size of a saucer between the dressing and the belt. The lack of both specific knowledge about daily care and equipment to manage the ostomy severely restricted the physician's ability to provide adequate postoperative care or counsel. As a result, patients resorted to a number of self-imposed limitations. Dietary restrictions were very common. Many patients, in attempting to reduce frequent colostomy spillage and enjoy a comfortable life, irrigated their colostomies with as much as 20–25 quarts of water, spending 24–56 hours a week at the task. Nevertheless, the lack of water-tight adhesive caused almost constant soilage of clothing. The resultant offensive odor produced profound feelings of horror, shame, and degradation in the patient; depression was common and often frankly suicidal.

Patients tended to be very secretive about their ostomies. Feelings of personal inadequacy and a morbid body image led many to seek separate beds or bedrooms, resulting in isolation within the family unit. Unfounded fear of injuring the altered internal body structure and the misguided belief that surgery had severely weakened the body prevented many patients from returning to their regular full employment. The resulting loss of earning placed additional stress on an already explosive situation. Not surprisingly, therefore, when Dyk, Sutherland, and their colleagues* evaluated the psychological

*Sutherland AM, Ohbach CE, Dyk RB, Bard M: Psychological impact of cancer and cancer surgery, Cancer 1952; 5:857–872; Dyk RB, Sutherland AM: Adaptation of spouse and other family members to the colostomy patient, Cancer 1956; 9:123–138.

impact of cancer and cancer surgery on patients who had undergone abdominoperineal resection for rectal cancer, they found that limited employment opportunities, restricted sexual activity, and severe alterations in social relationships within the family and community had created a nightmare for most ostomates.

Fortunately, several aspects of treatment have changed in recent years, all to the benefit of the patient. Since the early 1950s when Bricker, Brooke, Crile, and Turnbull introduced new surgical techniques, we have seen numerous advances in the surgical construction of ostomies. At the same time, the appliances and equipment available to manage them have improved tremendously, and much more advice is now available for patients.

The many advances in ostomy construction, equipment, and management are very welcome. However, unless this information is made readily available to members of the health team caring for patients with cancer and to the patients themselves, the horrors of life with an ostomy that Dyk and Sutherland described in the late 1950s will be as prevalent today. Excellent textbooks on ostomy care have been published recently, we realize, but most are encyclopedic in scope and none focuses on the special needs of patients with cancer.

We have, therefore, undertaken this challenge: to make more accessible the knowledge about ostomy construction and ostomy care for patients who are also burdened with cancer treatment. We have written this book for every member of the health care team—the surgeon, the internist, the nurse, the enterostomal therapist, and others who participate in caring for the patient. We have tried to present the basic considerations of ostomy care and those that are unique to patients with cancer, including special complications caused by chemotherapy or radiotherapy. In examining potential problems we offer methods that have led to useful solutions for us.

Our ultimate goal has been to make rehabilitation attainable for our special group of patients. It is our hope that this work will help patients to return more readily to their usual daily activities—whether at work, with their families, or in their social lives.

*Dorothy B. Smith*
*Douglas E. Johnson*

# Acknowledgments

This book represents a compilation of the disappointments and accomplishments of the many who have labored in the past, the direct and indirect contributions of scores of dedicated professionals working in the present, and our hopes for the future; as a result, we are indebted to many. We wish particularly to express our deep appreciation to our contributors for their willingness to share their expertise in such a wide range of areas; without the input from multiple disciplines, care of the ostomy in a patient with cancer would be far from complete.

We are indebted to Gero von le Fort, head of Medical Illustration & Graphic Design at The University of Texas M. D. Anderson Hospital and Tumor Institute at Houston, to John Kuykendall and James Bibbins for the excellent photographs, and to Patricia Carlson for the superb illustrations. To Lonna Sager we extend special thanks for her untiring efforts in seeing the manuscript through all its various stages and endless revisions. In addition, we are most appreciative of our publishers, who provided us a means of communication.

No words can express our gratitude to Barbara Reschke, our medical editor, adviser, and friend. It was her efforts in taking the diverse manuscripts and polishing and blending them into a unified array that assured completion of this project in its allotted time.

Last and most important, we thank our patients. From the beginning, they have been an integral part of the team; they provided us our experience and gave us the meaning for our work.

*D.B.S.*
*D.E.J.*

# Contributors

Joseph N. Corriere, Jr., M.D.
 Professor and Director, Division of
 Urology
 The University of Texas Medical School
 at Houston
 Houston, Texas

Susan Dudas, R.N., M.S.N., E.T.
 Associate Professor
 University of Illinois College of Nursing
 Chicago, Illinois

David M. Gershenson, M.D.
 Associate Professor of Gynecology
 The University of Texas M. D.
 Anderson Hospital and Tumor
 Institute at Houston
 Houston, Texas

Stephen L. Huber, M.S., R.Ph.
 Assistant Director of Pharmacy
 The University of Texas M. D.
 Anderson Hospital and Tumor
 Institute at Houston
 Houston, Texas

Douglas E. Johnson, M.D.
 Ashbel Smith Professor of Urology
 The University of Texas M. D.
 Anderson Hospital and Tumor
 Institute at Houston
 Houston, Texas

Christopher J. Logothetis, M.D.
 Associate Internist/Associate Professor
 of Medicine
 The University of Texas M. D.
 Anderson Hospital and Tumor
 Institute at Houston
 Houston, Texas

Leslie R. Schover, Ph.D.
 Assistant Professor of Urology
 (Psychology)
 The University of Texas M. D.
 Anderson Hospital and Tumor
 Institute at Houston
 Houston, Texas

Dorothy B. Smith, R.N., M.S., E.T.
 Department of Nursing
 The University of Texas M. D.
 Anderson Hospital and Tumor
 Institute at Houston
 Houston, Texas

Stephen B. Tucker, M.D.
 Assistant Professor of Dermatology
 The University of Texas Medical School
 at Houston
 Houston, Texas

Gunar K. Zagars, M.D.
 Assistant Professor of Radiotherapy
 The University of Texas M. D.
 Anderson Hospital and Tumor
 Institute at Houston
 Houston, Texas

# Ostomy Care and the Cancer Patient

## Surgical and Clinical Considerations

Dorothy B. Smith
Douglas E. Johnson

# 1

# Preoperative Preparation

One of the most difficult periods for people who have cancer is the interval between the time they learn that they need an ostomy and the time they undergo the planned surgery. It is an emotionally labile period for patients and their families, a time full of fears, uncertainties, and questions. Nevertheless, if a patient is to be effectively rehabilitated, this preoperative preparatory period must be used to the maximum.

Rehabilitation is never accomplished through the work of one person, but requires the combined efforts of a team working closely together. This team begins with the patient and his or her family and includes the physician, nursing staff, social worker, and enterostomal therapist (ET nurse). During the early preoperative preparatory period, the members of this health care team have the responsibility to assess all patients' capabilities carefully and to identify any limitations that may affect their ability to cope with stomal care. At the same time, the team must foster in patients and their families a positive attitude toward caring for the proposed ostomy. Between them, the team members must see that each patient understands what the stoma is and what it involves. In addition, they must select the proper location for the ostomy. Since Chapter 5 discusses patient teaching in detail, we focus in this chapter on patient assessment, patient attitudes, and stoma site selection.

## PATIENT ASSESSMENT

The primary goals of patient assessment are to determine the patient's capabilities for satisfactorily managing the proposed ostomy and to identify any adverse factors that can be modified to make ostomy care easier. Obviously, a person who has been only marginally able to care for himself, to work, or to engage in social life may be incapable of assuming the responsibility for ostomy care. Likewise, the presence of physical handicaps may limit a person's ability to care for an ostomy. Therefore, the health care team must make every effort to evaluate thoroughly each patient's capabilities, to review carefully the methods of home care presently operative, and to establish realistically what tasks a patient can master through lessons in the hospital.

Patients should never be stereotyped as "confused," "depressed," or "slow" or labeled with other prejudicial terms that may limit their chances of being given a fair opportunity to learn to care for themselves. Although sometimes the challenge for the staff may be larger and the demands for patience greater, the goals remain the same in every instance: to provide the most effective treatment for all patients while at the same time enabling them to return to *their* way of life.

We cannot overemphasize the importance of patient assessment. It is like a double-edged sword. On the one hand, if exenterative surgery

THE CANCER PATIENT WITH AN OSTOMY
ISBN 0-8089-1807-9

offers the most effective means of eradicating the malignancy but a patient is deemed incapable of managing the ostomy, that patient may be denied the best chance for living; yet, on the other hand, if surgery is performed, the ostomy created, and the patient proves incapable of caring for the diversion, then the resulting quality of life may be so poor as to erase any benefits gained from the additional survival. We therefore offer the following suggestions for assessing a patient's mental, physical, and emotional status, hoping to help members of the health care team arrive at the correct decision about the patient's ability to care for the ostomy and identify any factors that may present special problems.

**Mental Status**

What is the status of the patient's memory? Is it affected by age or anxiety? Does the patient have a learning disability or an emotional disorder? Each patient receives instruction about care of the stoma and appliances while in the hospital and is expected to assume these responsibilities at home; obviously, the patient must have the requisite learning faculties.

If the health care team has questions about a patient's ability to learn, additional time for instruction should be scheduled before surgery, either in the clinic or in the hospital, before the patient's mind is clouded with postoperative pain and narcotics and his or her energy drained from the surgical insults. We guide such patients through the basic steps of ostomy care, making sure that they are capable of performing each task.

Even though a patient may have someone at home who can assist with personal care, we make every effort to help patients achieve personal independence. It is a terrible burden for a patient not to be able to empty a pouch or change it, should a leak occur.

**Physical Status**

Total physical condition, of course, determines whether patients are acceptable risks for surgery. In deciding whether a patient will be able to care for an ostomy, however, the health care team must pay special attention to manual dexterity and visual acuity. They also need to be attuned to other factors that could adversely affect the ease with which a patient learns to cope with an ostomy. In order to teach effectively and to select appropriate equipment, therefore, they should seek information about each patient's hearing, skin sensitivity, and life activities.

In extreme situations, either visual impairment, lack of manual skill, or loss of hearing may necessitate altering the type of urinary or fecal diversion that the surgeon has in mind. A continent ileostomy (Kock pouch), which does not require an external appliance but, instead, periodic catheterizations, may be a solution for a patient with physical disabilities. Occasionally, when a patient is unable to care for an external appliance at all, a continent proctostomy or some type of colocystoplasty or ileocystoplasty must be substituted for an external ostomy. Only a complete physical evaluation can determine when one of these options must be employed.

*Dexterity*

Does the patient have a tremor? Has it been evaluated previously, and can it be controlled or reduced by medication? Does the patient have arthritis involving the fingers? Has he had a stroke with residual immobility? Is he missing fingers? A hand? An arm?

When manual dexterity is in question, to know what a patient can do with his hands becomes imperative. Can he hit a nail with a hammer? Can she sew, knit, or make a quilt? Will the patient be able to open the drain valve or clamp the drainage tube of the ostomy pouch, peel off the adhesive backing, or apply a pouch on a faceplate? One way to find out is to have the patient practice preparing and applying an appliance.

The patient's degree of dexterity frequently influences the selection of appliances. A one-piece, precut appliance is much easier to work with than a two-piece appliance. Painting surgical cement on the pouch may be easier than applying an adhesive disc. These are just some of the many alternatives that a nurse may have to try to see which will prove best for the person who has problems with dexterity.

*Vision*

Visual ability seriously affects ostomy care. Occasionally, one has to abandon the idea of constructing an ostomy because the patient can-this occurs rarely. Recently we taught a mentally alert blind 93-year-old male to apply a one-piece presized three-inch Hollister pouch over his transverse loop colostomy by touch. He learned to close the clamp by placing it in the same position between his fingers each time and pressing the release valve with his thumb.

In assessing the patient's visual abilities one should ask whether he reads a newspaper. Does he wear glasses? Are the glasses bifocal or trifocal? (Sometimes looking down at a specific spot on the abdomen through trifocals is difficult.) When we are unsure about vision, we mark a circle on the patient's abdomen, have him or her stand, and ask him or her to put a faceplate or pouch on the mark. Standing and looking ahead into a lighted magnified make-up mirror allows some patients to see the mark when they otherwise could not (Fig. 1-1). If vision is significantly impaired, patients may be taught to apply the appliance by touch, using the stoma as a landmark for setting the appliance on the abdomen, as we taught our elderly blind patient. Alternatively, patients can compensate for errors in centering the pouch opening over the stoma by slightly enlarging the opening in the appliance. Although this results in incomplete skin protection, it is preferable to traumatizing the stoma or allowing frequent leakage of urine from an off-center appliance.

*Hearing*

We rarely think of hearing loss as a problem in ostomy care, but when it is severe it can be a frustrating impediment to learning. Elderly patients who have lost hearing gradually through aging become very adept at socializing and conversing without revealing the degree of their hearing loss. Consequently, members of the health care team must be alert to evaluate what a patient is interpreting. They must make sure that their patient is understanding the message and not just agreeing with everything they say. A good way to check what patients are hearing and learning is to ask them to repeat in their own words what the teacher has said; another method is to require them to perform a new task after they have received the necessary verbal instructions. Written and visual instructions are helpful in teaching all patients, but they become especially important when a patient has a hearing loss. After their discharge from the hospital

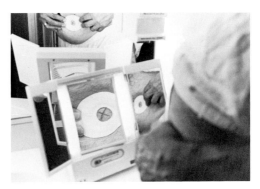

**Figure 1-1.** A lighted make-up mirror may provide enough magnification to allow a patient with poor vision to see the potential stoma site.

is too late to learn that patients have not heard the instructions for ostomy care.

*Skin Problems*

Does the patient have any localized or systemic skin disorders? Are they located in areas where the stoma would normally be located? Is the skin fair, dry, oily? Will the skin characteristics affect the ostomy seal?

The development and general availability of hypoallergenic appliances, skin adhesives, etc., have eliminated many of the problems with skin care that we encountered frequently a decade or so ago. However, occasionally one still sees a patient whose skin is intolerant of almost all appliances. It is imperative, therefore, that the health care team be cognizant of the patient's allergic history. If it seems severe, the team should consider preoperative patch testing and even, in some cases, encourage the patient to wear various appliances preoperatively; these means should identify any intolerances prior to surgery.

## Life Activities

As the health care team members evaluate patients' physical status, they must determine how they interact with their environment both at work and at home. How is the patient employed? What does he or she like to do for recreation or hobbies? The answers to these simple questions may provide important information about the most appropriate kind of ostomy, the patient's ability to learn and to care for himself or herself, and any special equipment needs.

The patient who sits in an air-conditioned office all day at work and reads for a hobby does not place the same demands on a urinary appliance or a colostomy pouch as a lineman who climbs telephone poles, a farmer who rides a tractor, or a retired teacher who plays golf, swims, and gardens for recreation. If the person works or plays outside in the heat, adhesives and skin barriers that melt are not suitable.

The information about life activities gathered at this time not only affects the choice of stoma and appliance, but also provides an activity baseline, enabling the health care team to evaluate the patient's rehabilitation by comparing preoperative activities with those the patient engages in after recovering from surgery.

## PATIENT ATTITUDES

Once we have determined that a patient is a suitable candidate for ostomy surgery, every member of the health care team becomes obligated to see that the patient and the family develop a positive attitude toward the ostomy and its care. Every team member's goal must be to return the patient to his or her usual activities after recovery from surgery.

Patients' initial reaction to, or attitude about, the proposed surgery and the ostomy reflects whatever prior information or misinformation they have acquired. Their immediate response may stem from total ignorance or from an experience with a family member or a friend who had an ostomy. Their knowledge may be limited to the memory of an old uncle who had a complicated urinary diversion procedure and was constantly wet, smelled terrible, and eventually died; or a grandmother who had a colostomy and, during her remaining days, was relegated to a back room. It is important to inquire about what patients may know; one can ask if they have ever known someone with an ostomy or have heard of a urinary diversion, a colostomy, or an ileostomy.

For teaching to be successful, patients and families must start with correct information. A planned approach usually begins with the physician discussing the disease, the proposed plan of care, and the type of surgery that will create the ostomy. Providing patients and families with literature about the disease, the surgery, and the ostomy helps them because it allows them to review and discuss the information together after the initial emotional shock has passed. If information is provided only verbally, anxiety may interfere with patients' understanding or their memory of what they hear. Patients should never be given literature without some explanation, however. In addition, the physician and nurse should allot some additional time a day or two later to allow patients and their family members to ask the questions that arise after they have had time to digest the information.

Immediately after they learn that they need an ostomy, patients are usually in a state of emotional shock. This is not a good time for learning. It is a time for the health care team to offer support, answer questions, and try to reduce the patients' anxiety.

Once patients have absorbed some of the shock of the news of the diagnosis and necessary surgery, however, they are usually interested in gathering information. This is a most opportune time to begin the teaching-learning process and to help patients formulate positive attitudes. At this time a second member of the health care team—a nurse or an ET, perhaps—reinforces information initially provided by the physician. He or she can reiterate or interpret what the physician said about the patient's disease, why this particular treatment has been selected, and how the surgery and ostomy may affect sexual function. The team member can describe the ostomy in detail—its construction, care, and the appliances needed—and can answer questions.[2]

Answering questions clearly and factually may be one of the most important functions the health care team performs, and well worth the time it takes preoperatively. During the question-and-answer process patients and families can clarify their ideas, and the health care personnel can assess their level of understanding. All team members who provide answers should listen carefully to patients, understand what they are really asking and the fears that lie behind the questions, and be supportive of the patients' concerns.

The questions we are asked most frequently before surgery are: can I wear my normal clothes? will I need a plastic sheet for the bed? can I return to my work? will my partner still love me? can I still travel (play golf, fish, hunt, swim)? will the pouch show through my clothing? can I feel my bowels moving? how will I go to the bathroom? how will I know when to empty the pouch? how often does the pouch need draining? can I bathe? what do I do about the urinary drainage at night? how do I keep the pouch from smelling? what can I do with the pouch during lovemaking? can I still have a beer? a martini?

We have found that using simple diagrams or drawings helps patients to visualize the planned surgery and how the ostomy is created. We use language that creates a visual image of what to expect for patients and their families. For example, we tell patients that the stoma will look and feel like the inner lip or cheek. Patients can touch and see the inside of their cheeks, and the comparison evokes a positive feeling. This is needed to counteract the negative connotations that accompany thinking of the stoma as a portion of the bowel. We try to convey to patients that the lining of the intestine is similar to the lining of the mouth and cheek, and consequently the stoma will be beefy red and moist like the inner lip. We explain that, when a patient first sees the stoma, it will be fastened around the edges with small sutures or staples, but that it will grow to the skin as it heals. Patients learn that they can care for the stoma much as they care for the rest of the abdomen, can bathe or shower with no special precautions, and can leave the appliance on or take it off, depending on whether they plan to change the pouch. For example, if, on a given day, a patient wants to change the pouch he can remove it, shower or bathe, then apply a new pouch. Or, if the pouch is securely in place and needs no changing, he may leave it on while he bathes or showers.

We have found that patients appreciate the opportunity to see and handle an ostomy appliance during the preoperative instructional period. We may not know exactly which appliance a patient will use postoperatively, but most pouches are similar in design, and seeing one gives the patient some idea of its size and the fit on his or her abdomen.

During the preoperative preparatory period, patients are building confidence in their physicians, the general nursing staff, the ET nurse, the social worker, and other members of the health care team. They are developing attitudes—either positive or negative—about the proposed ostomy and whether they can learn to care for it themselves, about body image and whether they will be less of a person after surgery, and about their ability to return to work, resume their usual social activities, and assume their previous roles in the home. Patients feel that they have little control over their lives at this time, and as a result are very vulnerable. It is important, therefore, that the staff work together, reinforcing each other's teaching, so that each patient perceives organization, confidence, and coordination preoperatively in the plan of care.

## STOMA SITE SELECTION

Although the total rehabilitation of the patient with an ostomy requires the interactions of multiple factors, proper placement of the stoma is the single most important one. This is the factor that determines whether the patient can wear an appliance securely and will be able to resume a normal life-style. Serious errors can be made in stoma site selection if this function is not included as part of the patient's preoperative preparation but, instead, is left to be determined arbitrarily at the time of surgery.

Although various writers have suggested that the ideal location for a stoma is a point midway between the umbilicus and the iliac crest, or at the center of a triangle created by the pubis, umbilicus, and iliac crest (Fig. 1-2), these specifications should be considered as only rough guidelines that usually have to be modified because of preexisting scars, folds, and other irregularities.[1,3–7] In selecting a stoma site, the physician should choose, first, an area that the patient can see, and second, one that provides a large smooth surface free of scars and wrinkles to support the faceplate and appliance. One should avoid bony prominences such as the iliac crest or costal rib margins, skin folds or creases, surgical scars or incisions, and existing hernias.

Since one's abdominal wall characteristics vary as one changes position, a patient must be examined not only when lying down, but also when sitting and standing. Infrequently, an area that appears perfectly satisfactory when the patient is prone becomes most unsatisfactory when he or she sits or stands, (Fig. 1-3) because of such factors as skin retraction resulting from an old surgical scar, shifting flesh beneath a protuberant belly, or, in women, large pendu-

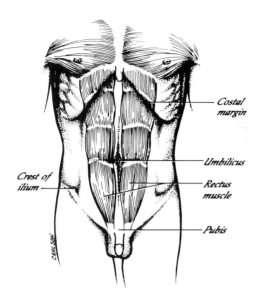

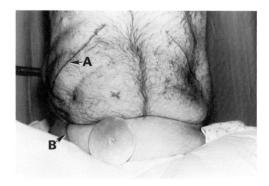

**Figure 1-3.** A patient being measured with marking discs for a urinary diversion. The costal margin (*A*) and iliac crest (*B*) have been identified and marked in black ink. The patient has a significant midline crease when he is sitting that must be avoided. The largest surface area available to support an appliance is identified by the marking disc.

**Figure 1-2.** Major anatomic landmarks that aid in selecting a stoma site.

lous breasts. When all factors are equal, the preferred site overlies the rectus abdominis muscle, which provides firm support for the faceplate. However, the cardinal rule of selecting a site with the greatest surface area should never be compromised in order to place the stoma over the rectus abdominis muscle. We have experienced no problems when the stoma either overlay the lateral margin or was totally outside the margins of the muscle.

Other factors may alter stoma site selection, such as prior radiation therapy, use of a lower-extremity prosthesis or back brace, and fear of compromising the blood supply to the wound in patients with prior paramedian incisions. When a patient has been irradiated, the surgeon should try to place the stoma outside the fields of therapy to minimize the problem of delayed healing and the increased risk of cellulitis brought on by the reduced vasculature of the tissue. Knowing the type of treatment and the fields employed is helpful. Unless this information, accompanied by pictures or descriptions of the radiation fields, is readily available from the patient's medical records, it should be requested from the radiotherapist. Careful examination of the abdomen, looking for any skin or subcutaneous tissue changes, is mandatory. Frequently,

when cobalt therapy or low-energy radiation has been used, the skin has darkened and the underlying tissue feels "woody" or "indurated" from the resulting fibrosis. These areas must be avoided in selecting a stoma site.

If the patient uses a prosthetic device, abdominal support, or back brace, the stoma site should be selected while the patient is wearing it. Does the support or any of its straps cross the abdomen or interfere with the location of the stoma or appliance? If so, and the brace has been custom made or fitted for a specific medical reason, it may be necessary to consult its manufacturer to determine what options are available for stoma site selection, appliance modification, or both. Can an opening for the ostomy be made in it without weakening the support? Can a leather support strap be modified or reanchored to accommodate the ostomy appliance? Would it be wise to choose a site on the opposite abdominal wall, away from the prosthesis? These and other alternatives need to be considered before surgery, so as to place the stoma properly and assure continued use of the prosthesis or brace.

An important factor in selecting an ostomy site, and one that is frequently overlooked, is the possible effect of the stomal incision on the blood supply to the operative wound when patients previously have undergone a paramedian incision, such as for an appendectomy. The surgeon should remember that the blood supply to the skin and underlying subcutaneous tissue runs obliquely downward from the posterior lateral direction toward the midline. When patients have already had a paramedian incision, the blood supply to the midline has been compromised. Consequently, when the surgeon excises a cancer through a midline incision and simultaneously creates an ostomy, the ostomy incision may severely restrict the blood supply to the major midline operative wound, resulting in poor wound healing, infection, and subsequent wound dehiscence. We have found this to be a special problem in obese patients and recommend that, at times, the surgeon strongly consider placing the stoma on the opposite abdominal wall.

If the patient requires the creation of two ostomies, as happens in a total pelvic exenteration requiring both a urinary conduit and a colostomy, the stomas must be located sufficiently far apart to allow appliances to be fitted over each. Whenever a patient needs both urinary and fecal stomas, we prefer to place the urinary stoma slightly higher to reduce the risk of infection and to prevent the belt of the urinary appliance (if needed) from overriding the colostomy stoma. This placement, however, is not always possible. Sometimes either the extent of the disease or the lack of available bowel to bring to the surface may dictate a less preferable location for the stoma.

In selecting a stoma site for a patient with cancer, it is wise to remember that the patient may require additional stomas in the future; sufficient areas for their placement should be available as the need demands. A patient who has undergone an anterior exenteration for bladder or cervical cancer and has a urinary conduit may later require a colostomy if cancer recurs in the pelvis. A patient with ovarian cancer who requires a bowel diversion may, at a later time, need other bowel bypass procedures for intestinal obstruction. Consequently, when choosing a stoma site the surgeon should be careful to select a location that does not jeopardize future treatment options.

Should any questions arise regarding the suitability of the stoma site that has been se-lected, patients should apply and wear an appliance before surgery, preferably both during the day and at night. They should be active—bending, sitting, walking, and twisting. We place a small amount of water in the pouch to determine if and from where the appliance leaks. If a leak occurs, we note where the adhesive seal broke by examining the back of the adhesive to see which point became wet. We must then select a new stoma site and check its suitability by again having the patient apply and wear an appliance. Although this procedure is time consuming, it is preferable to finding out postoperatively that the stoma is in a position that will not support an appliance and leaves the patient constantly soiled.

Once the proper stoma site has been selected, the physician should mark it so that subsequent bathing and surgical skin preparations will not remove it. Several indelible-ink pens are available for stoma site marking, but we prefer to be absolutely sure: we mark the site either by scratching an "X" in the skin, using a sterile 25-gauge needle, or by injecting intradermally a minute amount of methylene blue. The disadvantage of this latter method is that, should the site not be chosen in surgery, the dye remains in the skin for a long period.

## CONCLUSION

An ostomy permanently changes the bodies of people with cancer, but it need not also change their way of life, provided members of the health care team plan and implement a systematic rehabilitative procedure.

Patients' postoperative adjustment is directly influenced by their ability to care for themselves, their attitudes toward the ostomy, and the placement of the stoma. These factors are the responsibility of the health care team. Therefore, between the day patients learn an ostomy is necessary and the day the surgery is performed, the team must carefully assess every patient, encourage positive attitudes, select the most appropriate site for the stoma, and begin teaching self-care.

By using this preoperative period fully and effectively, the health care team can start their patients on the road to independence, thus preventing a lifetime of unnecessary frustration.

## REFERENCES

1. Greer B: Guidelines for stoma construction. Ostomy Management, May-June, 1978, pp 3–6
2. Hernandez M: Preoperative considerations for the ostomy patient. Cancer Bull 33(1):6–8, 1981
3. Kodner IJ: Colostomy and ileostomy in clinical symposia. Ciba Found Symp 30(5):1–35, 1978
4. Lerner J, Eisenstat TE, Spear J: Pitfalls of Stoma Placement. Baltimore, Departments of Surgery and Nursing, University of Maryland Hospital, 1981, pp 1–8
5. Smith DB: Stoma site selection. J Enterostom Ther 9(6):60–64, 1982
6. Turnbull RB Jr, Weakley FL: Colectomy and ileostomy for ulcerative colitis: location of the stoma and the abdominal incision, in Atlas of Intestinal Stomas. St. Louis, C. V. Mosby, 1967, pp 7–9
7. Watt RC: Stoma placement, in Broadwell D, Jackson B (Eds): Principles of Ostomy Care. St. Louis, C. V. Mosby, 1982, pp 329–339

Douglas E. Johnson
Dorothy B. Smith

# 2

# Urinary Diversions

The number and variety of urinary diversion procedures developed over the past 100 years attest to the ingenuity of surgeons in trying to devise the most satisfactory and universally acceptable procedure. It is unlikely, however, that any single procedure will ever satisfy the needs of all patients, since the factors involved in selecting a urinary diversion are never quite the same. The choice of an operation requires very careful and critical appraisal. Mogg[80] has emphasized the five most important factors to consider: (1) the reasons for the diversion, (2) the condition of the available tissues, (3) the functioning state of the urinary tract, (4) the age of the patient, and (5) the patient's psychological reaction to the proposed new way of life. Two additional factors, not applicable to patients with benign disease, must be considered in selecting a urinary diversion for a patient with cancer. The first is whether the diversion is being performed for palliation or as part of a planned therapeutic program that is likely to be curative. The second, an outgrowth of the first, is whether additional cancer treatments (irradiation, chemotherapy, immunotherapy, alone or in varying combinations) are likely to be necessary and, if so, what impact they and the urinary diversion will have on each other.

Usually, a urinary diversion in a patient with cancer is created after a long and complicated exenterative procedure (radical cystectomy, anterior exenteration, or total pelvic exenteration) has been completed. Under these circumstances the diversion must be created quickly, without placing additional stress on the patient. In addition, since the most common malignant diseases requiring exenterative surgery (colorectal, bladder, and cervical cancer) have a tendency to recur within the pelvis, the diversion should be constructed above the pelvis, if possible, to lessen the risks of obstructive problems should disease recur locally and to eliminate injury to the new urinary tract should irradiation to the pelvis be necessary postoperatively. Consequently, attempts to implant the ureters in the intact bowel or into an artificial bladder constructed from the stomach, the small intestine, or the colon are usually contraindicated. Furthermore, these latter diversion procedures carry with them increased risks for sepsis, especially if myelosuppressive chemotherapy is required at a later date. The surgeon who is considering a permanent urinary diversion procedure for a patient with malignant disease is usually limited in his or her choices, therefore, to a cutaneous ureterostomy or some type of urinary conduit. These procedures have proven to be the simplest and most expedient to construct, have the greatest likelihood of early primary healing, and are accompanied by the fewest early and late complications.

## CUTANEOUS URETEROSTOMY

### Historical Development

Gigon of Angouleme,[33] in 1856, was the first to suggest the use of ureterostomy to reestablish drainage in a patient with an obstructed ureter.

Unfortunately, his treatment recommendations for a patient with bilateral ureteral calculi were ignored and the patient died of anuria. Twenty-five years later, Gluck and Zeller[34] successfully performed cutaneous ureterostomy in dogs, and a few years after that Laurenze,[66] in Rome, brought to the skin a ureter that he had accidentally cut.

Le Dentu[68] is the man who should be credited with deliberately using cutaneous ureterostomy for supravesical urinary diversion. He chose the procedure in 1889, in an attempt to relieve anuria in a woman with uterine cancer whose ureters had become involved by the pelvic malignancy. By bringing the left ureter to the skin above the iliac crest he established free drainage, although the patient died from carcinoma within two weeks. In 1895 Wassiljew[115] first employed ureterocutaneous transplants in conjunction with cystectomy; later, in 1939, Hinman and Smith,[48] reviewing all the experience with total cystectomy reported in the literature, noted that cutaneous ureterostomy had been chosen as the method of urinary diversion for almost a quarter of the patients.

Even though the distal end of the ureter sloughed frequently, requiring reoperation, and suitable urinary appliances were unavailable, a third of American urologists were still using cutaneous ureterostomy in preference to implantation into the bowel as late as 1955.[23] However, during the late 1950s, as surgeons gained experience with the recently introduced ileal conduit, they began abandoning routine cutaneous ureterostomies for the more satisfactory intestinal conduit. Today, cutaneous ureterostomy for cancer patients is restricted to highly selected situations.

## Indications

Cutaneous ureterostomy is a satisfactory and effective method of providing drainage for the upper urinary tracts when restricted to patients with a chronically dilated ureter or ureters. The procedure is especially applicable as a means of temporary diversion in infants and young children with such diverse conditions as ureteral valves, severe bladder outflow obstruction, megacystis syndrome, dysplasia of the abdominal wall muscles (prune-belly syndrome), and severely refluxing megaloureters,[27] but is indicated only occasionally for permanent ureteral diversion in patients with pelvic malignancies.

The operation has a low mortality, a minimal early morbidity, and causes no electrolyte imbalances. Its major advantages, especially for a patient with a solitary kidney, are the ease and quickness with which the diversion can be constructed. The procedure makes unnecessary the intestinal surgery that ileal and sigmoid conduits require, thereby either minimizing or eliminating the risks of intestinal anastomotic leaks, intestinal obstruction, and peritonitis.

The importance of selecting only patients with at least one chronically dilated ureter cannot be overemphasized. A thin-walled ureter, the result of an acute obstruction, is unsuitable. Surgical disasters may be expected when patients are selected who do not have a chronically dilated (thick walled), tortuous ureter with a well preserved blood supply.[9]

## Surgical Technique

To construct a safe and successful cutaneous ureterostomy, the surgeon must bring the ureter out to the skin in a direct fashion, without undue tension, allowing sufficient length to create a stoma of adequate caliber. Various types of cutaneous ureterostomies (Fig. 2-1) have been described,[2,45,65,69,111,116] but for patients with malignant disease we recommend only a transureteroureterostomy with a cutaneous ureterostomy or, if the patient has a solitary kidney, a unilateral cutaneous end ureterostomy. Bilateral cutaneous ureterostomy, resulting in two stomas that require two separate appliances, is not recommended and can be justified only in emergency situations that demand the rapid termination of surgery. A double-barreled ureterostomy in an adult requires an inordinate amount of ureteral length to locate the stoma in either iliac fossa and therefore can rarely, if ever, be constructed safely according to the tenets already outlined. We recommend against placing the stoma in the midline or umbilical region, because cancer patients frequently require additional abdominal operations. In addition, appliances are usually more difficult to apply in this location. It is imperative, as we emphasized in Chapter 1, that the site for the stoma be chosen carefully before surgery so that an appliance can be fitted easily and maintained postoperatively by the patient (Fig. 2-2).

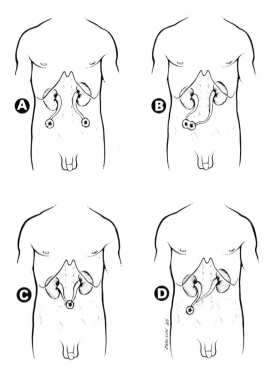

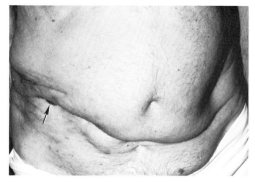

**Figure 2-2.** This 65-year-old man underwent a palliative urinary diversion for inoperable bladder cancer. No consideration was given preoperatively to selecting a stoma site, and at the time of surgery an end cutaneous ureterostomy was constructed (arrow). Note that the stoma was placed in an abdominal crease adjacent to the iliac crest and close to surgical scars. The man was referred for consultation when his local health care team could not fit him with an appliance.

**Figure 2-1.** Various types of cutaneous ureterostomy. **A**, Bilateral end ureterostomy. **B** and **C**, Double-barreled ureterostomy. **D**, Ureteroureterostomy.

The operation is usually performed through the transperitoneal route. After carefully completing an exploratory laparotomy and performing any additionally required surgical procedures, the surgeon mobilizes the ureter or ureters and places a suture in the distal end of each. Next, the surgeon should ascertain that the ureters are long enough so that the dilated ureter can be brought out through the proposed stomal incision in a retroperitoneal fashion and in an unobstructed, gentle curve. Our preference, as soon as we are sure of sufficient ureteral length, is to next develop the retroperitoneal tunnel. We excise a small button of skin and subcutaneous tissue down to the abdominal wall fascia, excise a small button of fascia, and develop a tunnel that will allow the ureter to pass unobstructed and without acute angulations to the skin surface. We then grasp the suture placed on the ureter and use it to pull the ureter out to the skin surface.

To perform a transureteroureterostomy

(Fig. 2-3), we bring the less-dilated ureter retroperitoneally across anterior to the aorta and vena cava to the site of the proposed cutaneous ureterostomy. Preferably, the ureter crosses the great vessels below the take-off of the inferior mesenteric artery. Next, we determine the proper location for the oblique end-to-side anastomosis of one ureter to the other. The anastomosis should be at least 1 cm long to allow for subsequent contraction. If possible, we excise a small window from the side of the dilated ureter to minimize the risk of a ureteroureterostomy stricture. We then place a posterior row of 4-0 chromic catgut sutures full thickness through the walls of both ureters, tying the knots on the outside. We pass a small Silastic stent through the incompleted end-ureterostomy up to the kidney and bring it out through the opposite ureter to the skin, where it is fixed with a 2-0 silk suture. A two-layer ureteroureterostomy anastomosis is constructed, using an inner layer of either interrupted sutures or running 4-0 chromic catgut sutures placed full thickness through both ureteral walls and an outer layer of interrupted 5-0 silk. A drain is brought out retroperitoneally through a separate stab incision some distance below the stoma, and the posterior peritoneum

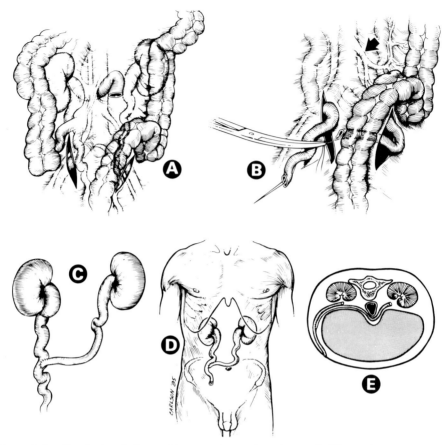

**Figure 2-3.**  Surgical technique of transureteroureterostomy. **A**, The ureters are exposed. **B**, The less-dilated ureter is brought to the opposite side in an avascular space in front of the great vessels, usually below the origin of the inferior mesenteric artery (arrow). **C**, The ureteroureterostomy is complete. **D** and **E**, Stoma is completed in the lower abdominal quadrant. Note the retroperitoneal location of both ureters.

is closed. We tack the ureter to the fascia with several interrupted chromic sutures and mature it to the skin without creating a bud, using interrupted chromic sutures.

Although we have not found a skin flap necessary in constructing the ureteral stoma, others[107,114] have recommended using it in hopes of preventing later scarring and contracture of the ureterostomy stoma.

### Complications

The major complications of cutaneous ureterostomy include necrosis of the stoma, retraction of the stoma, and stomal stenosis. These complications are directly related to the ureter's tenuous blood supply, which can be jeopardized easily by excessive ureteral mobilization, rough handling of the ureter by the surgeon during the operation, or constrictions compressing the ureter at the level of fascia, muscle, or skin. To reduce the likelihood of these complications, the surgeon must constantly exert meticulous care in handling the ureter throughout surgery. Preserving as much of the periureteral tissue as possible during ureteral mobilization helps to protect it. So does the fine catgut suture that should be placed through the distal end of the ureter, which provides the urologist with a "handle" to the ureter and minimizes the risk of crush injury from inappropriate use of tissue forceps. The retroperitoneal tunnel through which the ureter is brought should be spacious and should have no constrictions at any level that might interfere with the blood supply. Placing several interrupted, fine chromic sutures to anchor the ureter to the fascia prevents its retraction below the fascial level, should the ureter pull away from the skin owing to necrosis of the stoma. One should remember that decompression of the obstructed ureter causes the ureter to shrink in both diameter and length. This is why the mobilized ureters must be long enough that no tension exists at the skin level when the stoma is created.

Other complications that may occur include: (1) inadequate drainage, the result of ureteral obstruction or dysfunction; (2) pyelonephritis; and (3) calculus disease. Ureteral dysfunction resulting from lack of adequate peristaltic activity brought on by operative trauma or prolonged distention can be managed easily by temporarily inserting a catheter through the stoma. If the surgeon was not careful enough in creating the retroperitoneal or abdominal wall tunnel, the ureter may be kinked or obstructed by a scissoring effect at the fascial level. Again, inserting a catheter through the stoma establishes satisfactory drainage; rarely, one has to resort to placing a percutaneous nephrostomy with stenting from above. When this happens, a stent or small indwelling Foley catheter may be needed permanently. Since many physicians are not familiar with the care and management of these catheters, and since they must be changed periodically, we have been able to carefully train a member of the family (husband, wife, son, daughter, etc.) to change the catheter when it does not appear to be draining satisfactorily.

Eckstein[27] reported that, although the early results of cutaneous ureterostomy were satisfactory, over half the permanent cutaneous ureterostomies had to be converted to intestinal conduits within seven years because of stomal complications. Although we, too, have had to convert some cutaneous ureterostomies to intestinal conduits because of long-term complications, we are convinced that conversion should be needed infrequently when the procedure is performed in the carefully selected patient with malignant disease.

## URINARY CONDUITS

### Ileal Conduit

#### Historical Development

The development of the ileal conduit over 35 years ago and its rapid acceptance by the urologic community can be traced to three important factors.* First, although numerous operations had been devised, no method of urinary diversion had proven totally satisfactory. As late as 1936, a review of the literature by Hinman and Weyrauch[49] detailing cumulative experience with over 1000 operations in which ureterointestinal implantations had been performed revealed a mortality of over 50 percent when the patients implanted had malignant disease. Regardless of the type of procedure performed, intestinal and urinary infections and obstructions remained the most frequent complications. Second, total exenterative pelvic surgery was introduced between 1940 and 1950 to treat selected advanced pelvic cancers, which made it necessary to transplant the ureters into something other than the intact colon. Attempts at creating a continent urinary reservoir had generally been unsuccessful. Third, the first external appliance that could be attached to the abdominal stoma with a water-tight seal became available. In 1949 Bricker, one of the pioneers in pelvic exenterative surgery, was introduced to the Rutzen ileostomy appliance and used it successfully on two of his patients; in these two the cecum and ascending colon had been used as a reservoir following cystectomy, but the patients were constantly wet. According to Bricker, the results with this appliance were so gratifying that his whole approach to urinary diversion was immediately changed and, as a result, he constructed ureteroileal conduits for the next three patients having exenterations. The first report[10] detailing the experience of these three patients, who were followed for only a short period, appeared in *Surgical Clinics of North America* in 1950. Since then the operation has become the standard procedure for urinary diversion; it offers the best method of avoiding operative com-

---

* In researching this section the authors have drawn heavily from the comments outlined by E. M. Bricker.[11] The reader is encouraged to read this fascinating review for additional details.

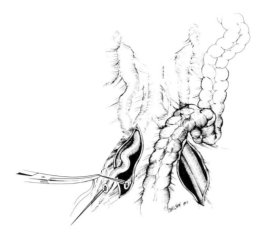

**Figure 2-4.** After developing a tunnel in the avascular tissue inferior to the sigmoid mesocolon, the surgeon brings the left ureter across in a gentle curve to lie on the right side.

plications, preserving renal function, and allowing the patient to live a relatively normal life.

We should emphasize, however, that Bricker was not the first to use the ileum as a means of urinary diversion. Zaayer,[119] in 1911, reported using it in two patients—in one to correct a vesicovaginal fistula caused by an invasive carcinoma of the cervix, and in the other as part of the treatment for an extensive bladder cancer. Unfortunately, both patients died within two weeks of surgery: one from her malignancy and the other from peritonitis. Later, in 1935, Seiffert[101] reported his results using a segment of jejunum in two patients, one of whom survived for longer than three years following cystectomy and urinary diversion for bladder cancer. In addition, during the same period in which Bricker was gaining his initial clinical experience with the procedure, Mersheimer and associates,[77,78] quite independently, were studying the problem in the laboratory in dogs.

*Indications*

The ileal conduit was developed for use in patients undergoing pelvic exenteration in whom intact bowel was not available for construction of either a ureterosigmoidostomy or some type of rectal bladder. Although it did not completely satisfy all the criteria for a successful urinary diversion, it did (1) reduce the likelihood of

recurring urinary tract infections by separating the urinary and fecal streams; (2) largely eliminate reabsorptive problems by serving as a transport mechanism for the urine, rather than a reservoir; (3) provide ready access for abdominal and pelvic surgery at a later date, if needed; and (4) allow the conduit to be inspected and the ureters catheterized endoscopically. Perhaps more important, it provided patients with a single stoma in a position they could easily manage. When one considers that the procedure was introduced in an era when all other methods available for supravesical diversion were generally unsatisfactory, one can readily appreciate why it gained such immediate acceptance. Today, with few modifications in the procedure as Bricker described it, the ileal conduit remains the most commonly used form of permanent urinary diversion.

*Surgical Technique*

In creating an ileal conduit, whether as a primary procedure or in conjunction with pelvic exenteration, the surgeon begins by identifying, isolating, and dividing the ureters near the pelvic brim. Both ureters are freed sufficiently so that they can lie in the right pelvis without tension. The surgeon must be careful not to strip the periureteral tissue too cleanly off the ureters. We temporarily ligate both ureters, although some surgeons[84] do not recommend the procedure, arguing that back-pressure can exacerbate possible preexisting urinary infection. However, we have noted no ill effects in the more than 500 patients in whom we have constructed conduits since 1968. Temporary ligation causes the ureters to dilate, thus facilitating suture placement at the time of the ureteroileal anastomoses. In addition, we can identify any segment of the pelvic ureter that does not dilate. When patients have received pelvic radiation, any segment that remains nondistensible and undilated should be suspect for radiation injury and should be excised at the time of the ureteroileal anastomosis.

Once the ureters are freed and relaxed, the surgeon bluntly creates a hole in the avascular tissue inferior to the sigmoid mesocolon between the superior hemorrhoidal artery and the sacrum. The left ureter is brought through this opening into the right pelvis in a gentle curve and without tension (Fig. 2-4).

The surgeon identifies the ileocecal junction and selects an approximately 15-cm long seg-

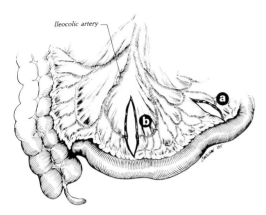

**Figure 2-5.** A segment of terminal ileum is selected and incisions are made in the mesentery. Note that the proximal incision (*a*) need not be as long as the distal incision (*b*).

ment of small intestine in the terminal ileum proximal to the ileocolic artery; this segment must be long enough to lie comfortably in the pelvis and to pass through the abdominal wall at the previously selected stoma site without tension. In estimating the length of ileum, it is preferable to err by making the conduit too long rather than too short; one can always shorten it later at the stomal end. Once the proposed segment has been selected, but before making any incisions, the surgeon must be sure that the mesentery to the proposed conduit is broadbased and has a good blood supply, as evidenced by its containing several complete vascular arcades. Transillumination of the mesentery helps to identify the vascular supply. The mesentery is then incised at right angles to the bowel axis at each end of the segment (Fig. 2-5). The length of the mesenteric incisions is determined partly by the thickness of the patient's abdominal wall and partly by the characteristics of the mesentery itself. The mesenteric incision made at the proximal or butt end of the conduit need not be as long as the one at the distal or stomal end. Once the mesentery has been divided, the mesenteric fat is cleaned from its ileal attachments for a distance of approximately 1.5 cm in both directions.

We prefer to divide the small intestine first at the proximal end and to close that end of the conduit before we divide the bowel at the distal end. This technique makes it impossible to construct a conduit other than in an isoperistaltic

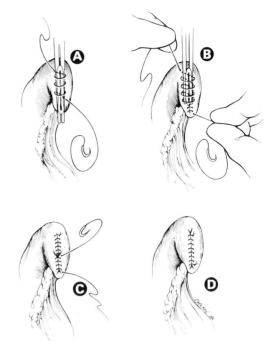

**Figure 2-6.** Closing the proximal end of the conduit. **A**, A running over-under stitch using 3-0 chromic catgut is placed. **B**, The noncrushing bowel clamp is removed and traction is applied to the ends of the suture so that the stitches are snug and the bowel walls are approximated. **C**, A second row of stitches is placed and the long ends of the sutures tied. **D**, An outer layer of inverting interrupted 3-0 silk Lembert sutures is placed to assure a water-tight anastomosis.

direction. If we plan to use sutures to reestablish continuity of the bowel, we apply noncrushing bowel clamps and divide the bowel between them; the proximal end of the conduit is then closed with an inner double layer of continuous 3-0 chromic catgut and an outer layer of inverting 3-0 silk sutures (Fig. 2-6). If, instead, we plan to reestablish bowel continuity by using stapling instruments, we apply the TA55 instrument to the proximal end of the conduit and a noncrushing bowel clamp adjacent to it. We then close the proximal end of the ileal loop with 3.5-mm long staples and incise the bowel over the TA30.

We next divide the bowel at the distal end of the ileal segment between noncrushing bowel clamps and place the loop caudad to the remaining small bowel. If the conduit is not in a caudal

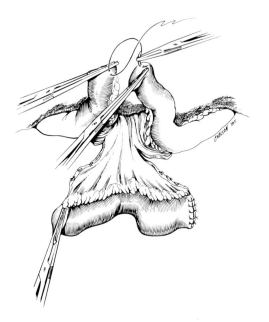

**Figure 2-7.** The first step in reestablishing bowel continuity is to place a row of posterior sutures close to the noncrushing bowel clamps.

position, it cannot be properly placed in the pelvis at the procedure's conclusion.

When bowel continuity is to be reestablished with sutures (Fig. 2-7), we perform a two-layer anastomosis, using 3-0 silk for both the internal and external layers. The two segments are held in close approximation and rotated slightly to expose the posterior bowel wall. A row of sutures is placed posteriorly as close to the clamp as possible, and the stitches at either end are left long to stabilize the bowel when the clamps are removed (Fig. 2-8A). A second row of posterior sutures is placed, beginning in the midline and moving from the center to the corner (Fig. 2-8B). Although many surgeons prefer a running chromic catgut suture for this internal layer, we prefer interrupted sutures because they provide a wider anastomosis. At the corners we use Connell stitches (inside-out; outside-in) to invert the mucosa; they are placed until they meet anteriorly in the midline (Fig. 2-8C). In placing these sutures, we have found it helpful not to cut the previous suture until the current stitch has been placed and tied; once a stitch has been placed, we bring the previous suture forward, turn the bowel inward, and tie the current stitch. When the bowel has been

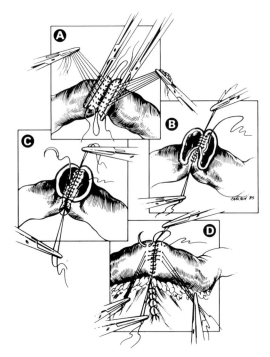

**Figure 2-8.** Technique for reestablishing bowel continuity.

joined anteriorly, restoring bowel continuity, we place in the anterior seromuscular coat of the bowel a row of interrupted 3-0 silk sutures similar to those placed earlier in the posterior wall (Fig. 2-8D). At this time we check the size and patency of the anastomosis by grasping the two ends of the bowel between a thumb and forefinger. Some physicians argue against this procedure, but we have found it helpful in assuring the surgical team that an adequate anastomosis has been created, and we have seen no ill effects as a result.

When bowel continuity is to be restored with the autosuture stapling technique (Fig. 2-9), we place several silk sutures into the bowel wall to maintain apposition of the two segments of ileum to be anastomosed; it is important to perform the anastomosis on the antimesenteric borders of the bowel. The two limbs of the GIA stapling instrument are inserted full-length into the bowel and locked in position. Two seromuscular 3-0 sutures are then placed at the end of the staple line while the bowel is steadied over the locked instrument. These sutures take tension off the staple line and prevent any "zipper"

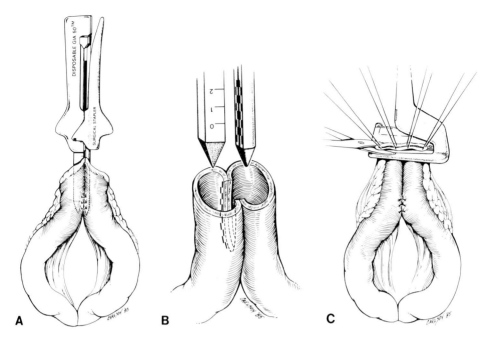

A    B    C

**Figure 2-9.** Autosuture technique. The GIA is locked in position on the antimesenteric border of the bowel and the knife is pushed forward, dividing the bowel between a double row of staples. **A**, Before removing the GIA, the surgeon places several sutures at the inferior margin to protect the stapled anastomosis from excessive traction, preventing a "zipper" effect. **B**, The instrument is removed and the staple line is inspected for luminal bleeding. **C**, The TA55 closes the common bowel lumen in one transverse application. Any excess bowel tissue is excised flush with the instrument before it is removed. The traction sutures shown help align the bowel edges in the jaws of the TA55.

effect. To make the anastomosis, the knife assembly is pushed forward and then backward. The two instrument limbs are unlocked, separated, and removed. The physician inspects the autosuture staple lines carefully to detect bleeding points; if any troublesome luminal bleeders are discovered, the physician controls them with a hemostatic suture of 3-0 silk.

The TA55 is used to close the common bowel lumen. Traction sutures are placed along the edges of the open bowel to facilitate accurate positioning of the instrument and to assure optimum placement of the staple suture line. One must take care to avoid face-to-face apposition of the luminal staple lines before applying the TA55. Care at this point should prevent the possible mucosal adherence and subsequent luminal obstruction for coaptation of the healing staple line, as reported by Elliot et al.[29] One transverse firing of the TA55 inserts a staple line that closes the bowel lumen. The surgeon ex-

cises excessive bowel tissue flush with the instrument before disengaging it from the closed bowel anastomosis.

Next, attention is directed to the ureteroileal anastomoses (Fig. 2-10). The left ureter is approximated to the antimesenteric portion of the proximal loop and fixed at that position with three 5-0 silk sutures, joining the periureteral and outer portions of the ureteral wall to the seromuscular layer of the bowel (Fig. 2-10*A*). Any excess ureter is excised at this time and the ureter is spatulated. A small button of the proximal bowel segment is excised at a location where the ureter can be easily approximated to it (Fig. 2-10*B*). The posterior end of the ureter is approximated to the small hole by three full-thickness 5-0 chromic sutures (Fig. 2-10*C*). A small Silastic ureteral stent is passed into the renal pelvis through the cut end of the ureter; the distal end of the stent passes through the intestinal segment. The anterior layer of the ureteroil-

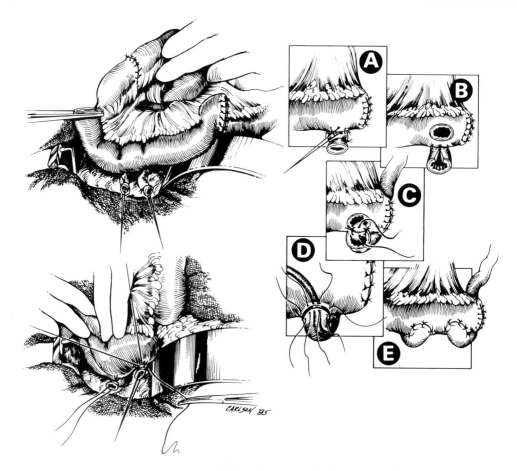

**Figure 2-10.**   Technique for ureteroileal anastomosis.

eal anastomosis is completed with additional interrupted full-thickness sutures of 5-0 chromic catgut (Fig. 2-10D). We prefer to have the knots on the outside and therefore place the sutures from outside the ureter to the inside and then inside the bowel to the outside. To complete the second layer, we suture the periureteral tissue to the bowel with 5-0 silk, making every attempt to assure a water-tight anastomosis.

After anastomosing the right ureter to the proximal intestinal loop in a similar fashion (Fig. 2-10E), we then prepare the stoma. We place Kocher clamps on the fascia of the anterior abdominal wall and pull all layers on the right side to the midline, so that they occupy the same position as they will when the incision is closed. This maneuver is imperative to avoid a scissoring effect on the ileal segment as it passes through the abdominal wall. A Kocher clamp is placed over the preselected stoma site, the skin elevated, and a 2–3 cm button of skin sharply excised with a knife (Fig. 2-11). Using electrocautery, we excise a plug of subcutaneous tissue down to the fascia and remove a small window of fascia. A large Kelly clamp, inserted through the fascia, points posteriorly away from the abdominal wall incision, tenting up the peritoneum. We incise the peritoneum and bluntly enlarge the opening in the fascia, rectus muscle, and peritoneum so that two fingers can be inserted easily.

The distal portion of the conduit, with the mesentery facing medially, is brought through the abdominal wall without tension (Fig. 2-12). The fascia over the rectus muscles is approximated to the seromuscular portion of the distal loop with interrupted sutures of 3-0 chromic (Fig. 2-13A). The surgeon must exercise care in

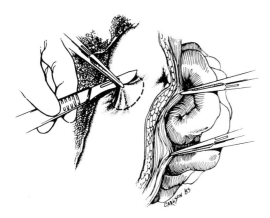

**Figure 2-11.** A circular skin incision is made over the preselected stoma site by elevating the skin with a Kocher clamp and incising sharply with the knife parallel to the body. Note that all layers of the abdominal wall have been pulled to the midline.

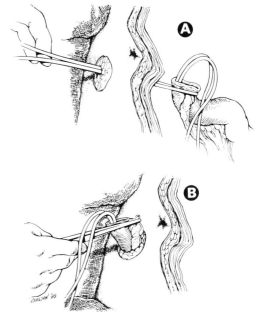

**Figure 2-12.** The conduit is brought through the abdominal wall (**A**) so that its mesentery lies in a medial position (**B**).

placing these sutures so as not to shorten the effective length of bowel between the fascia and the skin. If the sutures in the seromuscular layer are placed too far out on the bowel, stomal retraction will result. If the fascial defect is not closed adequately, however, a parastomal hernia may develop.

Next the bowel clamp is removed and the portion of the terminal loop that it has crushed is excised. The conduit is approximated to the skin with 3-0 chromic to create a flush (Fig. 2-13*B*) or nipple (Fig. 2-13*C*) stoma. The ureteral stents are fixed to the peristomal skin and cut so that they protrude 8 cm from the stoma.

After the stoma has been completed, the proximal end of the ileal segment is fixed to the left medial margin of the posterior peritoneal opening with several 3-0 interrupted silk sutures. Finally, before closing the wound, the surgeon closes the defect in the bowel mesentery with interrupted 3-0 silk sutures, taking care not to injure the blood vessels within the mesentery.

### Complications

The high operative mortality—ranging from 15 percent to 20 percent—reported during the late 1950s and early 1960s following construction of ileal conduits in patients with malignant disease has been significantly reduced over the last several decades. Today, the operative mortality

is in the range of 3–5 percent.[9,57] The infrequent deaths are usually the result of pulmonary emboli and myocardial infarctions, but occasionally result from sepsis originating in either the urinary tract, surgical incision, or lungs. Furthermore, the high incidence of wound infections (15–25 percent) recorded in earlier reviews[20,58,108] has decreased significantly in recent years, chiefly because of improvements in bowel preparation and the rational use of new antibiotics, administered parenterally in the perioperative period, which assure adequate tissue levels of appropriate drugs before the organisms can reach the wound. In spite of these improvements, however, both early and late complications occur in almost a third of the patients.

Complications may be expected in five major areas: (1) in the abdomen, either as a result of the route necessary for the surgery or as a consequence of the intestinal anastomosis, (2) within the kidney, (3) at the sites of ureteroileal anastomoses, (4) within the ileal conduit, and (5) at the stoma site.

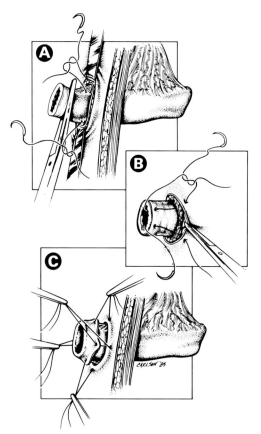

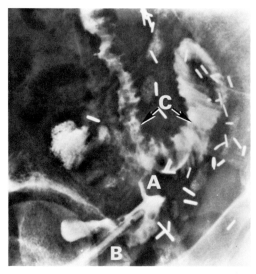

**Figure 2-14.**   A small intestinal fistula (*A*) at the site of an enterostomy was diagnosed by inserting a small catheter into the fistula tract (B) *and injecting contrast medium. Note that the medium passes readily into loops of the small bowel (C).*

**Figure 2-13.**   Technique for completing and maturing the stoma. **A,** The fascia is approximated to the bowel. **B,** The mucosa is sutured to the skin to create a flush stoma. **C,** The mucosa is everted to create a nipple.

*Intestinal obstruction.*   Paralytic ileus is normally present for 5–7 days following surgery and is readily managed by either a nasogastric sump tube connected to regulated wall suction or a gastrostomy tube, depending on the surgeon's preference. Certainly, a gastrostomy tube should be considered for any patient with compromised pulmonary function, since an indwelling nasogastric tube interferes with and restricts the patient's ventilatory efforts.

A mechanical bowel obstruction can develop at any time. It may result from adhesions that constrict a bowel segment or from internal hernias that occur most frequently either behind the ileal loop or through rents in the bowel mesentery. Less frequently, ischemic changes in the bowel produce a functional bowel obstruction that can mimic a mechanical obstruction. Late-occurring bowel obstructions are usually the result of recurrent malignancy.

Initial treatment should consist of passing a long tube (Canter, Miller-Abbott, etc.) into the bowel to remove the air and fluid and overcome the obstruction; while the tube is in place, the patient's nutritional status is maintained by intravenous hyperalimentation. Surgical intervention may be required to lyse adhesions and to correct specific causes of the obstruction.

*Intestinal fistulas.*   Intestinal fistulas, usually developing at the site of the enterostomy, have been reported in about 5 percent of patients (Fig. 2-14). Although our early experience with the autosuture stapling technique suggested its association with a slightly higher occurrence of fistulas,[56] neither the accumulated results in the literature[61,86] nor our own most recent experience suggests any significant difference in the incidence of anastomotic leakage attributable to the method used for reestablishing bowel continuity.

Late-occurring fistulas are usually the result of one or more predisposing factors: pelvic abscess, recurrent tumor, prior irradiation, or bowel obstruction. The small bowel's contents may discharge spontaneously through the vagina in women, through the urethra in men who have undergone cystectomy, or from an anterior abdominal wall phlegmon. On rare occasions, an ileal conduit enteric fistula discharges the small bowel contents from the ileal stoma.[89]

Treatment consists of establishing adequate drainage to the outside and, in the absence of distal intestinal obstruction, maintaining the patient's nutritional status; the fistula usually closes spontaneously. Occasionally, however, surgical intervention is required—either excising the segment of bowel involved or bypassing the fistula site and creating a mucous fistula.

*Pyelonephritis.* Acute pyelonephritis has been recorded as an early complication (occurring before the patient leaves the hospital) in about 3 percent of patients who receive urinary diversions. However, its incidence in all patients who have undergone ileal conduit construction increases as a function of the time the patients are under follow-up, and can be directly related to the incidence of ureteroileal anastomotic strictures, calculi, and residual urine in the conduit. Sullivan and associates[108] reported that over 19 percent of their patients followed for five years or longer had experienced at least one episode of acute pyelonephritis and that chronic pyelonephritis, as determined by radiographs, was evidenced in one-fifth of their patients at five years. This is not surprising, since the review of Gregory and associates[37] showed that 55 of 439 patients (13 percent), or 86 of 960 renal units (9 percent), investigated radiographically showed signs of postoperative renal deterioration. In their own series of 81 patients who survived five or more years after ileal diversion, these investigators found that 12 percent of the renal units had deteriorated when they studied them radiographically.

Treatment for pyelonephritis generally consists of, first, instituting appropriate parenteral antibiotic therapy, based upon urine culture and sensitivity reports,[106,117,120] and second, correcting, if possible, any predisposing factors (ureteral obstruction, calculus disease, etc.). Patients who have recurrent attacks of acute pyelonephritis (two or more per year) may benefit from oral antibiotics (cephalosporin, carbenicillin sodium) taken prophylactically, once a day, usually prior to retiring at night. Patients suffering with chronic pyelonephritis may need to be placed on a long-term suppressive antibiotic regimen.

*Calculi.* Stones form postoperatively in 6–12 percent of patients who have ileal conduit diversions, although a few series have reported an incidence as high as 30 percent.[38] Interestingly, stones appear at first glance to develop less often in patients with malignant disease (3–5 percent), but these figures probably reflect the fact that calculus formation is usually a late complication, seldom apparent within the first two years. In support of this thesis, Sullivan and associates[108] recorded only a 4 percent overall incidence of postoperative stones in their 336 patients with bladder cancer who underwent single-stage cystectomy and construction of an ileal conduit, but when patients remaining alive at five years were studied, the incidence had increased significantly to 15 percent, with the majority of the stones occurring in the left kidney.

Dretler,[24] studying the pathogenesis of urinary tract calculi occurring after ileal conduit diversion, concluded that pyelonephritis, urea-splitting organisms, high-conduit residual urine, and hyperchloremic acidosis were common in patients who formed stones and distinguished them from other patients who underwent diversion. He suggested the following mechanisms of pathogenesis: (1) excess conduit length or conduit dysfunction, which enhances chloride-bicarbonate exchange; (2) chronic bicarbonate loss, which creates a need for bone buffering and results in hypercalciuria; (3) hypercalciuria, which in the presence of an alkaline urine (from urea-splitting organisms and reflux of bicarbonate-rich urine) creates a favorable environment for calculus precipitation (Fig. 2-15). Treatment is similar to that for calculus disease occurring in patients without a urinary diversion.

Occasionally, calculi form in the conduit as a result of foreign bodies. When the proximal end of the loop has been closed by the autosuture technique, urinary salts can precipitate around an exposed staple.[3,5,7,43] Halverstadt and Fraley[39] have reported calculi forming also on a nonabsorbable silk suture used to anchor the base of the conduit retroperitoneally. The suture apparently had eroded into the loop and served as a nidus for stone formation. Giant calculi,

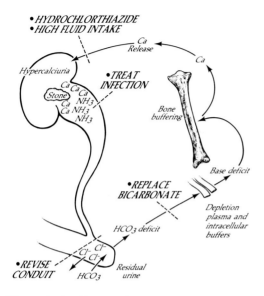

**Figure 2-15.** Proposed mechanism of calculus formation and possible preventive measures. (Reprinted with permission from J Urol 109:208, copyright 1973 by The Williams and Wilkins Co., Baltimore.)

usually the result of stomal stenosis and residual urine within the conduit, are encountered occasionally and may require stomal revision to remove them.

*Ureteral obstruction.* Stenosis of the ureteroileal anastomosis occurs in 6–18 percent of patients; again, the incidence reflects the length of time the patient has been followed since surgery. Sullivan and colleagues[108] noted that, within six months of surgery, 2 percent of patients developed ureteroileal strictures caused by fibrosis—1 percent on the right side and 1 percent on the left; however, the incidence increased progressively with time. When patients survived five years, 4.8 percent had strictures on the right, 8.3 percent had them on the left, and 2.4 percent had bilateral strictures. In addition, obstruction had developed as a result of intrinsic malignancy in 3.3 percent, extrinsic cancer in 1.8 percent, and ureteral calculi in 2.1 percent of the five-year survivors.

The management of ureteroileal anastomotic strictures depends upon many factors: (1) degree of ureteral obstruction, (2) status of renal function, (3) severity of symptoms (pain, fever, etc.), (4) physical condition of the patient, and (5) status of the malignancy. For a patient with a unilateral, asymptomatic ureteroileal anastomotic stricture whose renal function is satisfactory and shows no evidence of deterioration, we recommend observation. For selected patients who are symptomatic or show evidence of compromised renal function, we may consider placing a percutaneous nephrostomy and, a few days later, dilating the ureteroileal anastomotic stricture, using progressively larger indwelling ureteral stents passed over a guide wire in an antegrade direction. If the ureteral obstruction persists in spite of these maneuvers and the patient's condition prevents surgical correction, an indwelling catheter may be inserted in either an antegrade or retrograde fashion over the guide wire to allow drainage from below. This negates the need for flank catheters and allows urine to drain through the preexisting ileal stoma into the usual collecting device.[100,104]

If the guide wire cannot pass through the stricture and if the patient's poor general physical condition or progressing malignancy precludes surgical correction, we may need to leave the nephrostomy tube permanently in place. When this occurs, we have later dilated the nephrostomy tract and inserted an indwelling Foley catheter, which permits easier catheter changes. Usually, however, we perform open surgical repair of the anastomotic stricture, using one of several available techniques. We prefer not to detach the obstructed ureter, but instead, once we have mobilized the distal ureter, we perform a side-to-side anastomosis over an indwelling ureteral stent. We then meticulously construct a water-tight anastomosis and close the wound without drains.

*Urinary fistulas.* A urinary fistula develops postoperatively in 2–5 percent of patients. It represents a serious complication, as the subsequent mortality approaches 50 percent.[44,88] The condition should be suspected in any patient who develops nonhypovolemic reduction in urinary output, prolonged ileus, fever of uncertain origin, abdominal distention, or "watery" discharge from the surgical incision. The most reliable test to establish the diagnosis is the retrograde ileogram (Fig. 2-16). Almost all leaks occur at the ureteroileal anastomosis, but on rare occassions a midureteral leak may develop.[40] Although diabetes mellitus[88] and prior

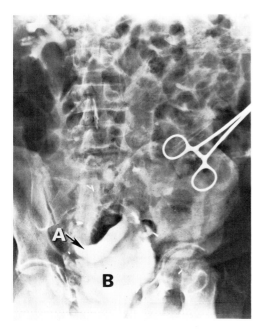

**Figure 2-16.** Retrograde ileogram showing a large leak, with extravasated contrast medium pooling in the pelvis. Note the ileal conduit (*A*) and the contrast medium present in the pelvis (*B*).

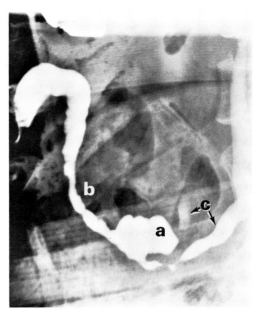

**Figure 2-17.** Ileal loop stenosis. A retrograde ileogram showing a normal proximal ileal conduit (*a*) but a stenotic distal segment (*b*). Reflux is evident in both ureters (*c*).

pelvic irradiation[21,32,88] have been suggested as predisposing factors, we believe that most cases can be directly attributed to surgical errors. When the surgeon handles the ureter carefully—preserving as much periureteral tissue as possible, excising all redundant ureteral tissue, and meticulously performing a two-layer water-tight anastomosis over an indwelling ureteral stent as previously described—this complication should very rarely, if ever, develop.

A leaking ureteroileal anastomosis does not necessarily require immediate surgical intervention, provided adequate drainage can be established. If the leak is small and the ureter remains attached to the ileal wall, percutaneous insertion of a ureteral stent in conjunction with a diverting nephrostomy may allow the fistula to heal without surgical correction. However, if the leak persists in the face of conservative measures for more than two or three days, the ureteroileal anastomosis must be repaired surgically.

*Ileal conduit stenosis.* Ileal conduit stenosis is an infrequent complication (Fig. 2-17).[30,41]

Mitchell and associates,[79] reviewing their experience with 12 instances, noted that the age of the ileal loop at the time the stenosis was diagnosed ranged from 4 to 14 years and averaged 9 years. Back pain and fever were the most common complaints. Radiation effect has been incriminated in some patients, but the cause of the stenosis is poorly understood. The pathogenesis appears to be a chronic inflammatory reaction causing progressive fibrosis in the mucosa and submucosa. A number of other factors have been suggested, including microvascular ischemia, urine-borne toxic material, infectious and allergic stimuli, and an immunologic defect.[41]

If the ileal conduit has narrowed diffusely, the entire conduit may need to be replaced. However, if the proximal segment is uninvolved and the ureteroileal anastomosis patent, then one may excise the distal stenotic and scarred portion of the conduit and use an add-on ileal loop, as described by Poor et al.,[95] to provide the necessary additional conduit length. This latter procedure avoids recreating the ureteroileostomy, with its inherent risk of ureteral leaks and obstruction.

*Parastomal hernia.* Parastomal hernia has been reported in between 2–10 percent of patients. Certainly, the frequency with which it is encountered can be directly related to the care exercised by the surgeon in obliterating the space between the conduit and the anterior abdominal wall fascia. A hernia may occur at any point around the conduit, but is most likely to develop medially, adjacent to the area where the mesentery exits through the fascia. Concern over injuring the blood supply to the conduit makes most surgeons fearful about placing secure sutures at this location, resulting in a potential space for a hernia to develop.

The need to repair a parastomal hernia is dictated by the symptoms it produces. Jaffe, Bricker, and Butcher reported only four of 543 patients with ileal conduits who subsequently underwent repair of a parastomal hernia.[52] Obviously, if the hernia is causing intestinal obstruction, pain, or problems in keeping the external urinary appliance in place, surgical correction is required. In at least one instance, a parastomal hernia mechanically obstructed an ileal conduit, causing total anuria.[71] However, if the hernia is producing no significant ill effects, it may be observed for the present, and surgically corrected only if symptoms develop.

A number of methods have been used to surgically repair parastomal hernias. In the uncomplicated case the repair is made by circumferentially incising the stoma at its cutaneous junction and freeing the conduit from its subcutaneous tissue attachments. The hernia sac is identified and carefully dissected; it is then returned to the abdominal cavity and the fascial defect is reapproximated, using nonabsorbable sutures. A large defect may require that the stoma be moved to a new site.[74] Occasionally, in complicated cases, Marlex mesh may be needed to reinforce or replace the fascia.[51]

*Stomal stenosis.* Stomal stenosis that requires operative intervention, caused by alkaline encrustation, hyperkeratosis, and peristomal scarring, has been recorded in as high as 50 percent of the children who undergo ileal conduit diversion.[25] Interestingly, in adults with cancer the incidence of stomal stenosis requiring surgical revision is only 2–6 percent.[14,90,109] We do not mean to imply, however, that all stomas in adults maintain their original size, only that not every adult stomal stenosis requires revision. In spite of the small size of some stomas,

stomal revision should be performed only when progressive obstructive uropathy, recurrent pyelonephritis, or calculus formation results from the stomal stenosis, impairing urinary flow.[109]

Many varied techniques have been described to correct stomal stenosis,[22,91,92,97] but by far the best treatment is prevention. The problem can usually be avoided if the surgeon pays careful attention to detail at the time the stoma is constructed and the patient wears a properly fitting appliance. The shape of the stoma seems to have no relationship to the incidence of stenosis. Some investigators suggest constructing either a bud stoma (see Fig. 2-13*C*)[55,75] or a Turnbull loop stoma[8] (Fig. 2-18) to minimize the occurrence of stomal stenosis, but we have seen no additional stomal problems with a flush stoma, our choice for several decades. We have relied on the flush stoma for over 450 patients with bladder cancer in whom we performed a radical cystectomy and ileal conduit diversion, and our incidence rate for stomal stenosis is 2 percent, similar to that in other reports.

*Miscellaneous.* Bleeding from an ileal conduit is an uncommon complication, occurring in only 1–2 percent of patients.[26] The bleeding most frequently is due to an ill-fitting appliance, but occasionally can be attributed to infection, calculi, tumor, or self-mutilation. Rarely has massive bleeding been reported.[73] Beaugie[4] and Hindmarsh[47] have reported fistulous formation between the conduit and iliac artery. Other causes for hematuria have included redundancy of the conduit resulting in stasis and infection,[59] Crohn's disease (regional ileitis) developing in the ileal conduit,[57,76,94] portal hypertension with formation of a "caput medusae" (Fig. 2-19),[26,31,70,118] and malignancy arising in the ileal conduit (Fig. 2-20).[64,103]

Rare complications reported with ileal conduits have included the development of adenomatous polyps within the conduit,[93,112] antibiotic-associated pseudomembranous colitis involving the ileal conduit,[102] acute ureteral obstruction secondary to mucoid impaction,[15] and volvulus of the ileal conduit, causing anuria.[63]

## Jejunal Conduit

Difficulties in using ileum that had been heavily irradiated or in constructing an ileal conduit in patients who had extensive ureteral

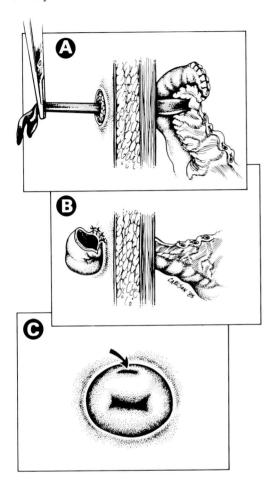

Figure 2-18. Loop-end ileostomy (Turnbull loop stoma). **A**, The proximal end of the conduit is closed, and an umbilical tape or small Penrose drain is passed through a small opening in the mesentery to pull the loop through the abdominal wall opening. **B** and **C**, After the loop has been anchored to the abdominal wall fascia, the conduit is opened transversely four-fifths of the way toward the distal end; both the proximal and the distal enterostomies are matured to the skin edge. The distal end (arrow) becomes a mucous fistula.

disease interfering with peristalsis led Clark[18] and Morales and Whitehead[85] to substitute jejunum for ileum. The additional length and the position of the jejunal mesentery provide greater flexibility for stomal placement; in addition, the longer jejunal segment is useful for replacing the varied lengths of ureter that may need to be excised due to disease.

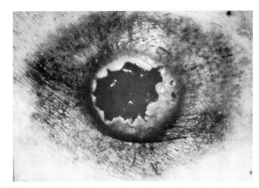

Figure 2-19. A caput medusae developing in a patient with portal hypertension.

The surgical technique for constructing a jejunal conduit is similar to that for an ileal conduit. The exact location and length of the jejunal segment to be isolated obviously depend upon the disease present and the patient's body habitus. After the surgeon has isolated the segment, he or she should place it medially before restoring the continuity of the bowel. The surgeon then closes the proximal end of the jejunal conduit and completes the enterostomy, using one of the techniques described previously for an ileal conduit. The ureters are brought through separate stab incisions in the posterior parietal peritoneum below the ligament of Treitz near the proximal end of the conduit, a two-layer watertight, refluxing, end-to-side, ureterojejunal anastomosis is constructed, and the stoma is created in a fashion identical to that for the ileal conduit.

Originally, physicians believed that the jejunum would not absorb urinary contents as

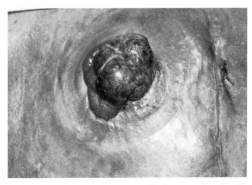

Figure 2-20. A tumor nodule is erupting in the ileal conduit.

much as the ileum did and therefore would be a highly satisfactory alternative for urinary diversion. In clinical practice, however, they found that almost half of the patients with a jejunal conduit developed, on one or more occasions, severe electrolyte disturbances: hyponatremia, hypochloremia, intracellular overhydration, hypovolemia secondary to jejunal excretion of water, extracellular hypoosmolarity, and azotemia.[17,35] The clinical manifestations of this syndrome consisted of anorexia, nausea, vomiting, and a moist tongue; cramps; various pains; personality changes; weakness; and occasionally convulsions or coma. To prevent these problems, patients must add salt to their diet. Because of the potential seriousness of these problems, jejunal conduits should be selected only when other forms of urinary diversion (ileal or colonic conduits) are impractical.

## Colonic Conduit

### Historical Development

It is impossible to identify any specific person or persons who should be credited for either conceptualizing or constructing the first sigmoid conduit. Without question, however, Mogg[81,82] deserves recognition for popularizing the procedure and for its acceptance as one of the surgeon's options for urinary diversion. Mogg's interest in using a defunctioned portion of the pelvic colon as a urinary conduit was first aroused in 1952, when he performed a staged radical excision of the rectum, prostate, and bladder, implanted the ureters into a loop of descending colon, and established a transverse colostomy in a 39-year-old man with rectal cancer. The patient lived in comfort for three years until he died of metastasis to the liver. After achieving a similar success in 1957 with a colon conduit in a four-year-old child with exstrophy and rectal prolapse, Mogg adopted the procedure exclusively as a means of diversion whenever a conduit was required in children.

When, in the late 1960s, the long-term results of ileal conduit diversions in children began showing a high incidence of complications, especially stomal stenosis and renal deterioration, the urologic community turned to the nonrefluxing colon conduit as an alternative to the refluxing ileal loop. Early results of the procedure were promising, but the long-term results

have shown no advantage to either children[28] or adults[72,110] for colonic conduits in place of ileal conduits; today, therefore, the choice of conduit is left to the discretion of the surgeon.

### Indications

Early proponents of the sigmoid conduit suggested that it had two major advantages over the ileal conduit: (1) less frequent stomal stenosis because of the larger diameter of the colon, which allowed for a larger cutaneous stoma, and (2) less deterioration of renal function, because it eliminated ureteral reflux by providing an intestinal wall that could allow antireflux ureteral anastomoses. Over time, however, longterm studies proved that these complications occurred no less often than in patients with ileal conduits. Consequently, indications for constructing a colonic conduit today are generally the same as for an ileal conduit, and the surgeon, in choosing a segment of intestine for constructing a conduit, should be influenced more by the operative findings and nuances of disease than by any attempt to reduce the long-term complications that are common to both types of diversion.

Specifically, a colon conduit is indicated for patients in whom prior injury or disease (radiation damage, regional enteritis, etc.) has affected the ileum, precluding its use, and for patients in whom disease or injury to the ureters requires the greater mesenteric mobility afforded by the colon to construct ureterointestinal anastomoses without tension. An additional indication for selecting a colon conduit is a total pelvic exenteration. By eliminating the need for a small bowel anastomosis in these patients, the operative time is reduced and potential anastomotic complications are eliminated.

### Operative Technique

*Sigmoid conduit.* The surgeon selects a 15- to 20-cm segment of the sigmoid colon, being careful to assure an adequate blood supply based on the inferior mesenteric artery. The sigmoid colon is mobilized from its lateral and posterior attachments and, at times, from the sacral promontory. If the sigmoid mesentery is not of sufficient length, the splenic flexure may also be mobilized to provide adequate length for the colocolostomy.[36] Once the sigmoid mesentery has been freed, the surgeon should be able to rotate the proximal conduit in either direction

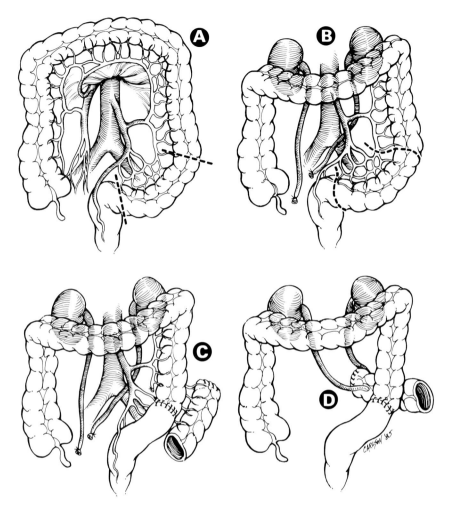

**Figure 2-21.** Isolation of the sigmoid colon. If additional mobility is required, the superior hemorrhoidal branch of the inferior mesenteric artery may be sacrificed.

so that, regardless of which side of the abdomen has been selected for the stoma site, the stomal (distal) end is in an isoperistaltic direction. In determining the length of the segment, the surgeon must remember that the isolated colon loop has a tendency to contract in length; he should therefore err in the direction of a too-long segment, which can always be shortened when the stoma is matured.

The surgeon makes the mesenteric incisions and, if additional mobility is required, divides the superior hemorrhoidal branch of the inferior mesenteric artery as he or she lengthens the inferior mesenteric incision (Fig. 2-21). Noncrushing clamps are applied to the proximal bowel, and the bowel is incised. The proximal end of the segment is closed, using a technique similar to one described for constructing an ileal conduit. The distal or stomal end of the segment is then incised between noncrushing clamps. The sigmoid loop, which has now been isolated, should remain above the bowel to be reconstituted if a right-sided stoma is to be created, or should be placed below for a left-sided stoma. Obviously, if a pelvic exenteration has been performed, bowel continuity need not be restored, and the sigmoid conduit can be placed in either lower abdominal quadrant, as the situation demands.

The surgeon restores colon continuity with

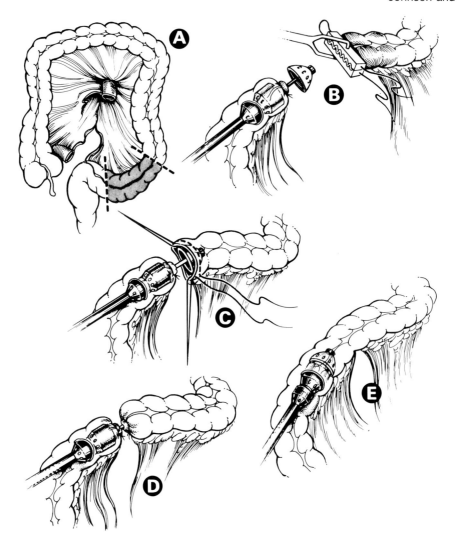

**Figure 2-22.** End-to-end anastomosis. (**A**) The site for isolating the sigmoid segment is identified. (**B**) Purse-string sutures are placed in the proximal and distal bowel segments. The placement of these sutures may be facilitated by using the special instrument as shown; a Keith needle has been introduced through the ends of the jaws. A proximal colotomy has been performed, the EEA stapler inserted, and a purse-string suture tied about the stem. (**C**) The anvil-nose cone is inserted into the distal lumen. (**D**) The distal purse string is tied tightly around the spindle. (**E**) The EEA instrument is fired, creating an end-to-end anastomosis.

a standard one- or two-layer closure similar to that described for constructing an ileal conduit. If he prefers, he may use the autosuture stapling technique, employing the EEA stapler to make the closures as described by Nance[87] (Fig. 2-22). When the EEA instrument is used, the surgeon carefully places purse-string sutures of 2-0 polypropylene monofilament in both the proximal and distal ends of the bowel to be anastamosed. This may be done either by hand or using the purse-string instrument, although the latter may be difficult to employ in the pelvis. The surgeon inserts the EEA autosuture instrument, with anvil attached, through a proximal antimesenteric colotomy and passes it through the proximal purse-string suture, which is then carefully tied over the spindle. Next, he passes the instrument beyond the distal purse-string suture, which is similarly tied. He then closes the instrument, approximating the bowel ends with the mesenteric borders properly aligned, and fires the instrument to create an end-to-end anastomosis. Afterwards, he partially opens the instrument and withdraws it, first through the anastomosis and then out the colotomy. The colotomy is closed in either one or two layers with sutures or with the TA55 autosuture instrument, as previously described. Last, the mesentery is reapproximated with sutures.

The next procedure is to mobilize the ureters. If they have not been previously detached as a result of pelvic surgery, they are incised close to the bladder. When a left-sided stoma is to be constructed, the right ureter is brought under the reanastomosed colon in a gentle curve to lie on the left side. The ureters are then anastomosed to the bowel, using the technique originally described by Leadbetter and Clarke[67] (Fig. 2-23). For the right ureter, the site of anastomosis is selected in the center of the taenia, close to the proximal or butt end of the loop. The surgeon makes an incision through the serosa and longitudinal muscle for a distance of approximately 5 cm. By blunt dissection the seromuscular flaps are raised on each side, wide enough to bury the ureter without causing obstruction (5–10 mm). Although it is preferable to develop a trough in a longitudinal muscle layer, where troublesome bleeding is less likely to occur, one may accidentally develop it in the submucosal plane; if that happens, less lateral dissection is needed.

The surgeon bevels the ureter, excises a small button of mucosa, and performs a mucosa-to-mucosa anastomosis using interrupted sutures of 4-0 chromic catgut placed through the full thickness of the ureter and the mucosa. Either immediately before placing the first suture or after tying several, we pass a small Silastic stent up the ureter to the renal pelvis and out through the sigmoid loop. We believe these tubes facilitate the placement of the sutures for the mucosa-to-mucosa anastomosis and prevent any obstructing sutures being taken through the

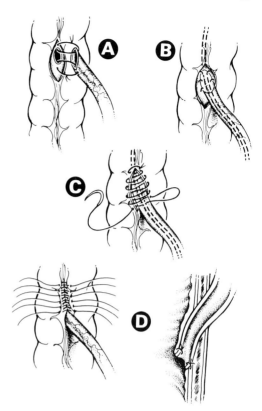

**Figure 2-23.** Ureterosigmoidostomy. **A**, A 5-cm incision is made in the taenia, close to the proximal end of the conduit, through serosa and longitudinal muscle. After a small button of mucosa has been excised, the proximal and distal margins of the ureteral lumen are sutured to their respective margins of the bowel lumen. **B**, The mucosa-to-mucosa anastomosis is complete. **C**, First-layer closure of the trough over the ureter. **D**, Second-layer closure of the trough.

opposing ureteral wall. We then approximate the flaps of the trough over the ureter, using either a continuous or interrupted suture of 4-0 chromic catgut. It is important to leave a liberal opening at the proximal end of the trough so as not to constrict the ureter. In placing the last suture, we include a small bite of the adventitia of the adjacent ureter, as described by Holden and Whitmore,[50] so as to telescope the ureter distally into the trough. This maneuver helps to maintain the trough at full length, to increase the length of ureter that lies within the trough, and to reduce

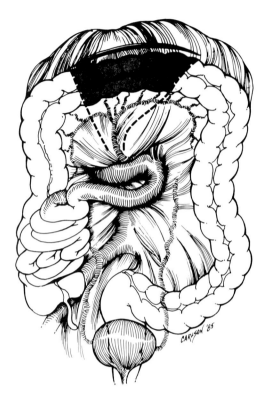

**Figure 2-24.** Mesenteric incisions that isolate a transverse colonic conduit.

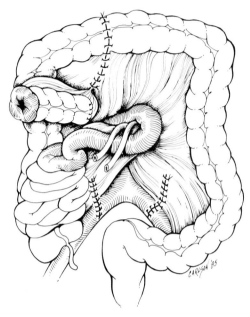

**Figure 2-25.** A transverse colon conduit is positioned near the root of the mesentery inferior to the colocolostomy. After both ureters have been isolated through separate incisions in the posterior peritoneum, they are brought into the peritoneal cavity through separate stab incisions near the butt of the colon conduit.

the tension on the mucosa-to-mucosa anastomosis.

We perform the left ureterocolonic anastomosis in a similar fashion at a slightly more distal position. After completing the ureterocolonic anastomoses, we create the stoma in a fashion similar to that described for the ileal stoma.

*Transverse colonic conduit.* A segment of transverse colon suitable for a conduit is usually shorter than the segment isolated for either an ileal or a sigmoid conduit. Nevertheless, the surgeon should be careful to select a segment that easily reaches the preselected stomal site in the anterior abdominal wall. He isolates the segment with a short proximal mesenteric incision to protect the blood supply and a longer distal incision to provide the necessary mobility for reaching the stoma site (Fig. 2-24). He divides the mesentery, as previously described for an ileal conduit, and cleans both the mesentery and appendices epiploicae from the serosal surface of the transverse colon for a distance of

several centimeters. Morales and Golimbu,[83] in describing the construction of a transverse colon conduit, have emphasized the importance of taking extra care so as not to injure the transverse mesocolon. The transverse colon is connected superiorly by the gastrocolic ligament of the greater omentum to the greater curvature of the stomach. To permit mobilization, this ligament must be detached from the transverse colon, but if one is not observant, one can easily encroach on the transverse mesocolon at this time.

Noncrushing bowel clamps are applied, and the proximal colon is detached and closed as previously described for an ileal conduit. Next, noncrushing bowel clamps are applied to the distal end and the colon divided. As described for a sigmoid conduit, the surgeon must be careful to place the conduit inferiorly before reestablishing bowel continuity. The proximal end of the colon conduit is attached to the posterior parietal peritoneum over the midline with interrupted 3-0 silk sutures (Fig. 2-25).

The next steps are to locate the ureters

through separate incisions in the posterior peritoneum, to dissect them free from their loose areolar attachments, and to mobilize them craniad, almost to the level of the renal pelvis. They are brought into the peritoneal cavity without twisting or angulation through separate stab incisions made next to the butt end of the colonic conduit, close to the ligament of Treitz.

In place of a Leadbetter, or antirefluxing, type of ureterocolonic anastomosis, as described for a sigmoid conduit, we construct an end-to-side, free-refluxing anastomosis similar to one described for ureteroileal anastomoses. After incising any redundant or ischemic ureteral segment, we fix the right ureter to the bowel close to the proximal end with several 5-0 silk sutures. We excise a small button of serosa, bowel wall, and mucosa and perform a two-layer ureterocolonic anastomosis, using a technique similar to that described for the ileal conduit. The ureter may be placed in the taenia, but this is not mandatory. Once the ureterocolonic anastomoses have been completed, we create the stoma, using procedures identical to those described for sigmoid and ileal conduits.

### Complications

The complications that follow the construction of a colonic conduit are similar in kind and frequency to those of ileal conduits.[46,83,110] For a description of their types and management, the reader is referred to the previous discussion.

Even though the early results of sigmoid conduits, as reported by Mogg[81,82] and others thereafter, were promising, longer-term follow-up studies have revealed more complications. Comparative studies[72,110] evaluating the results with those of ileal conduit diversions show similar complication rates for the two procedures and demonstrate no advantage for the colon, except in cases of total pelvic exenteration.[60]

Recently, Chiang et al.[16] reported the first occurrence of adenocarcinoma developing in a colon conduit, raising the concern that, as follow-up becomes longer, the incidence of malignant disease developing in colonic conduits may increase. Colon cancer has been calculated to occur 500 times more often in a patient with a ureterosigmoidostomy than in the normal population and constitutes about a 5 percent lifetime risk.[96,113] If a similarly significant association emerges between carcinoma of the colon and

colon conduits, more cases should begin to appear in the late 1980s.

## CARE OF THE STOMA

The care of a cutaneous ureterostomy and a conduit urinary diversion, both postoperatively and long term, are essentially the same. The stoma of a cutaneous ureterostomy may be smaller and, because of either the length of the ureter or the tenuous blood supply to the stoma end, may be retracted, but the principles of appliance selection and skin care are the same for both types of diversion; accordingly, we discuss them as one.

### Immediate Postoperative Care

Immediately after the surgery, in either the operating room or the recovery room, the ostomy is fitted with a urinary appliance.[53] This provides a means of collecting urine to monitor output and protects the skin from irritation. In the early postoperative period we usually prefer a clear disposable urinary pouch and skin barrier.[19,98] The skin barrier can be applied directly over sutures and can be custom cut to fit snugly around the stoma. The disposable pouch can also be custom cut to the stoma size, and has the advantage of allowing the nurse and surgeon opportunity to monitor the color of the stoma, patency of the stents, and urinary output. There are several types of skin barriers and pouches that can be used postoperatively (Fig. 2-26).

To prepare the skin around a new stoma, we wash it gently with warm water and pat it dry, being careful not to put tension on the new sutures or to cause bleeding. If the sutures are still oozing blood, we apply gentle pressure with gauze for a brief period.

We prefer to use a synthetic skin-barrier wafer of gelatin and pectin and a separate pouch, because they can be adapted to various sizes of stomas and are flexible enough to fit near or over an incision if necessary. We cut the opening of the wafer to the exact size of the stoma (Fig. 2-27).

We then choose a pouch that is clear, flexible, and has a urinary drain adaptor. The opening in the pouch may be $\frac{1}{16}$-inch to $\frac{1}{8}$-inch larger than the stoma because the skin barrier fits snugly and protects the skin (Fig. 2-28); an

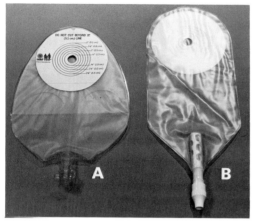

Figure 2-26. Disposable clear urinary pouches useful postoperatively (*A*, United; *B*, Marten). They may be custom cut and can be used with a skin barrier.

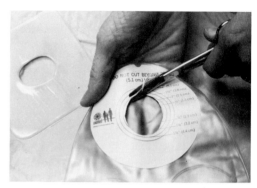

Figure 2-28. The adhesive backing of the pouch is cut $\frac{1}{8}$-inch larger than the stoma.

antireflux panel is desirable, to keep the urine from washing back up over the stoma.

We then apply the pouch to the skin barrier wafer (Fig. 2-29). Some doctors prefer a snap-on wafer and pouch system that allows the pouch to be removed for stoma observation without disturbing the skin barrier (Fig. 2-30). For their patients, we cut the wafer like a skin barrier, presize the pouch opening to match the wafer ring, and apply the pouch to the skin barrier or wafer, making it a one-piece unit, before we put it on the patient. This reduces the chance of leakage between the wafer and the pouch.

Just before applying the pouch, we recheck the skin to see that it is still dry and then remove

the adhesive backing from the skin barrier. If stents are in place, we insert a finger into the pouch opening and push out the back side of the pouch to make room for them (Fig. 2-31).

We pinch the stents to momentarily occlude the flow of urine, slide them into the pouch, center the pouch opening over the stoma, and gently press the adhesive to the skin. If urine is leaking around the stents, it may be easier to place the top half of the pouch on the dry skin first to position the pouch correctly, and then to raise the lower half of the adhesive to dry the skin before quickly pressing the adhesive to the skin.

The first data about the stoma should be recorded at this time. Included are the color of the stoma; its size; whether it is nippled, flush, or retracted; the presence, patency, and number of stents; and the condition of the skin.[99] These notes provide a basis for comparison so that

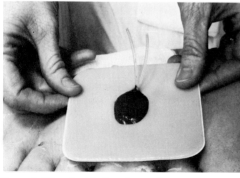

Figure 2-27. A skin-barrier wafer custom cut to fit snugly around the stoma.

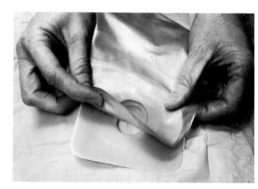

Figure 2-29. The pouch is attached to the skin barrier and the unit can be applied as one piece.

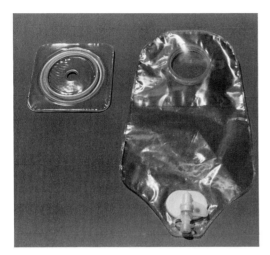

**Figure 2-30.** A two-piece unit (Conva Tec) that allows the pouch to be removed without disturbing the skin barrier.

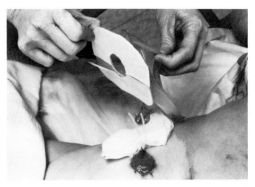

**Figure 2-31.** The back side of the pouch is pushed out to make room for inserting the stents. A gauze is used to catch any urine that may be spilling from the stoma while the stents are slid into the pouch.

other persons examining the stoma can detect changes or early signs of problems. Early postoperative problems to watch for are stoma necrosis, bleeding, suture separation, retraction, sloughing, skin irritation, and stent occlusion.[42] Bleeding that is not controlled by pressure, one or more sutures separating, occlusion of a stent, or ischemia of the stoma are serious problems that need immediate attention.

We leave a disposable postoperative pouch on our patients for five to seven days, changing it every second or third day, until they have recovered somewhat from the immediate effects of surgery and can begin to learn how to care for the stoma themselves.

### Choosing Permanent Equipment

As the patient recovers from surgery, the nurse begins to plan the type of urinary equipment that will be most suitable for the individual patient at home. The appliance selected must provide firm support at the base of the stoma, prevent urine from undermining the adhesive, provide a secure seal, wear comfortably, and be easy to apply.[12]

Several factors must be considered when selecting the type of equipment for the patient to wear at home. First, one must determine the characteristics of the stoma itself. Is it flush, protruding, or retracted? Next should be an examination of the patient's abdomen. Is it flabby or hard? Scarred? Has radiation induced changes in the skin? Where does the beltline occur?

Location of the stoma is a particularly important factor. Is it near a bony prominence? Is it in the beltline, or in a skin fold, or near a scar? Is it located in close proximity to another stoma, or horizontal to another stoma? Location in any of these sites can create problems for the patient, which a carefully selected, well-fitted appliance may help to solve.

Two other groups of factors should be evaluated before determining the most suitable appliance for a given patient. The first is related to the personal variables of the patient: his or her size, manual dexterity, and visual acuity. What type of work does the patient perform? What style of clothing does he or she prefer? What are the patient's financial resources, and what appliance can he or she afford? The final applicable factor concerns the appliance itself: what kinds are available where the patient lives? For a partial list of manufacturers of disposable and reusable appliances, see Appendix 2-1.

Urinary appliances are made in two basic types, disposable and reusable (Fig. 2-32).[105] Table 2-1 summarizes and compares their characteristics.

When measuring a stoma for a reusable appliance, one should plan the opening of the faceplate to be large enough so as not to cut or rub the stoma and small enough to keep the urine from continually contacting the skin (Fig.

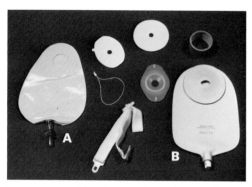

**Figure 2-32.** Two types of reusable appliances: a two-piece with faceplate and pouch separate (*A*, United) and a one-piece with plate and pouch as a single unit (*B*, Perma-Type).

2-33). A general rule when measuring is to allow a $\frac{1}{16}$-inch border around the stoma. A flush or retracted stoma can be fitted more closely than a budded or prolapsed stoma because the latter runs a higher risk of potential trauma from the plate (Fig. 2-34).

Most commercial plates come in round increments of $\frac{1}{16}$ inch or $\frac{1}{8}$ inch. If the stoma is oddly shaped, the faceplate opening should match. Some commercial plates are made of materials that can be adapted by a knife or a drill, so a special pattern can be made. Custom-made faceplates can also be ordered for stomas that are not uniformly shaped.

It is important to select a faceplate correctly sized by convexity as well as opening. The convexity of the plate should match the character of the stoma and of the abdomen. If the

**Table 2-1**
Characteristics of Urinary Appliances

| Advantages | Disadvantages |
|---|---|
| *Disposable* | |
| Lightweight | Not very durable |
| Low profile | Expensive |
| No cleaning necessary | Require adaptation if stoma not well made or properly sited |
| Can be purchased with pre-cut openings | Available only flat or slightly convex |
| Flexible | Melting skin barrier can occlude stent-guide openings and trap urine on the skin |
| Available for immediate purchase | Some of the skin barriers cause an odor when they react with urine |
| Convenient for travel | |
| One- or two-piece available | |
| Skin barrier built into some pouches | |
| Available with antireflux panel | |
| Require no additional adhesive | |
| *Reusable* | |
| Durable | Require cleaning |
| Moderate cost (up to ¼ the price of disposable*) | Heavier in weight |
| May be custom made for problem stomas | Waiting time necessary when ordering custom-made equipment |
| Deep convexity available | Require additional adhesive, either cement or disc |
| Proper fit prevents hyperplasia | Appliance material may absorb odor |
| One- or two-piece available | |
| Opening is pre-cut | |
| Pouches interchangeable among faceplates | |
| Antireflux panel available | |
| Nonadhesive appliance available | |

* Based on one year's appliance and adhesive cost (no skin products included) when pouches are changed twice a week.[13]

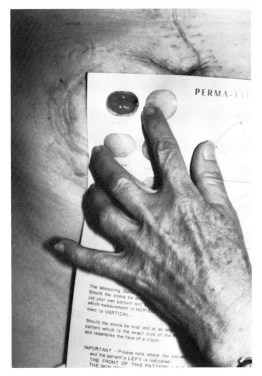

**Figure 2-33.** Measuring an oval stoma for a reusable appliance.

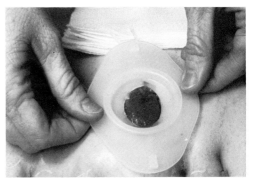

**Figure 2-34.** The faceplate should be approximately $\frac{1}{16}$-inch larger than the stoma.

the pouch to adhere to or when the surface becomes wet with urine very quickly. The cement, applied by a brush, is easier for some patients to manage manually. There are no openings to cut, no holes to align (as with the adhesive disc and faceplate), and no tape wrin-

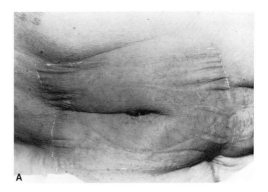

stoma is flush or nippled with no retraction, the plate can be flat. If the stoma is somewhat retracted or in a skin fold (Fig. 2-35A), the plate must have a convexity to match the degree of indentation (Fig. 2-35B). If the abdomen is soft, flabby, or filled with wrinkles, a firm plate is needed to stabilize the area, but if the abdomen is firm or muscular, the plate should be soft; a hard plate rocks on a firm abdomen. The rule of opposites applies: soft abdomen—hard plate; hard abdomen—soft plate.

Reusable appliances may be applied with either double-faced adhesive discs or surgical cement. Each has advantages and disadvantages. Double-faced adhesive discs can be purchased with presized openings cut to match the opening of the faceplate. They are easy to carry if an extra is needed, are not as messy to work with as cement, and are easier to remove from the faceplate. Surgical cement is a viscous adhesive that provides an immediate seal. Patients find it especially useful for solving problems, for example when there is very little surface area for

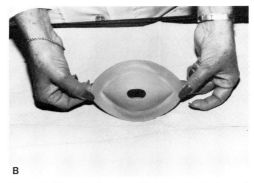

B

**Figure 2-35.** **A,** A stoma that is retracted and in a skin fold, creating a crease. **B,** The convexity of the faceplate must match the degree of retraction to prevent urine leakage along the crease.

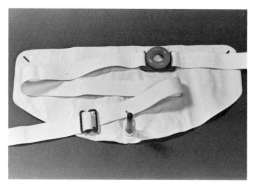

**Figure 2-36.** A nonadhesive urinary pouch that is supported by a belt.

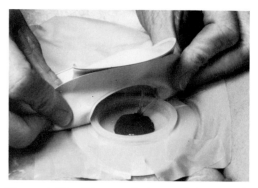

**Figure 2-37.** The pouch is applied over the extended lip of the faceplate.

kles to fuss with. However, cleaning the cement from the faceplate requires a solvent and is more time-consuming than removing an adhesive disc. One should consider these factors before deciding which method is most appropriate for a given patient.

If a patient has multiple skin problems from the adhesives or is not able to manually apply the adhesive-backed pouches, a nonadhesive urinary pouch may be the solution (Fig. 2-36). One is available that is held in place by a belt.[1,54,62] A soft ring inserted into the pouch opening is centered around the stoma. The belt is adjusted to fit the patient securely, and the pouch is buttoned on to it. Unlike adhesive pouches, which can remain in place up to seven days, this pouch should be removed daily. If the ring is left in place too long, it may cause a pressure ulcer to develop around the stoma.

Six to eight weeks after surgery the stoma must be remeasured, because its size changes as healing occurs and edema resolves. If a faceplate opening has become too large, it allows urine to constantly bathe the skin, causing irritation, hyperplasia, and *Monilia* infection (see Chapter 10).

Like fingerprints or noses, no two stomas are alike. No one appliance or manufacturer can fit every patient, and what works well for one patient may leak for another. Each person should wear the appliance that is best for him.

### Applying the Appliance

Immediately after surgery, members of the health team care for the urinary stoma, relieving patients of any responsibility for ostomy care.

But once the proper appliance has been selected and patients are able to concentrate on learning, we teach them self-care. Teaching may begin on the fourth or fifth postoperative day or it may begin later, depending on patients' rate of recovery from surgery. We start by explaining the procedure to patients, showing them what we are doing and preparing them for their role the next time the appliance is changed. We do not expect patients to learn everything in one lesson, but they can begin participating by actively preparing the equipment, learning part by part until the entire procedure is familiar. As we teach, we help patients to incorporate ostomy care into their own life-style and offer suggestions for managing at home (Appendix 2-2).

If a presized adhesive disc is not available, we trace a pattern from the faceplate onto the disc. We cut out the opening in the disc, and also cut four strips of waterproof tape approximately four inches long. We then remove one side of the backing from the adhesive disc, align the openings of the adhesive disc and the faceplate, and fix the adhesive on the disc, pressing down any wrinkles that may develop (especially on a convex plate). Then we remove the rest of the backing from the adhesive.

The next step is to clean and dry the skin. When it is ready, we center the faceplate over the stoma, press it to the skin for a few seconds, and then "picture-frame" the faceplate with the four strips of waterproof tape. To apply the pouch over the faceplate, we start with the bottom of the rim (Fig. 2-37) and hold the collar of the pouch, anchoring one side while pulling the other side. This should be done with gentle, steady motions, taking care not to dislodge the

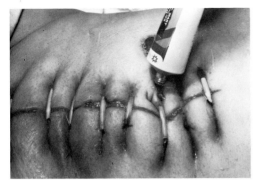

**Figure 2-38.** Skin barrier paste is used in small amounts to fill a crevice caused by a retention suture.

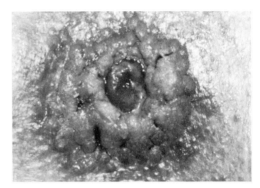

**Figure 2-39.** Hyperplasia around a urinary stoma that has been improperly fitted with an appliance, allowing urine continuously to saturate the skin.

plate. One can check the pouch by turning it. If it is not completely in place, it comes off the rim with the turn.

When all is secure, the pouch should be anchored on the faceplate with an elastic or tie and the pouch drain should be closed. If a patient would like to "dress up" the pouch, he or she can add a decorative pouch cover.

## Managing Problems

Good preoperative preparation, intraoperative technique, and immediate postoperative care can prevent many of the problems that plague patients with urinary diversions. Unfortunately, however, all stomas are not ideally located or constructed. Physicians and nurses who see only a few cancer patients with stomas each year are bound to run into problems with the stomas themselves, with appliance fit, and with patient facility that seem insurmountable. Following are some bits of practical advice for difficult situations.

When the stoma is located near a bony prominence, it can be fitted in one of several ways. Sometimes a pediatric-size faceplate is adequate. Another possibility is to use a plastic faceplate, trimming back the edge near the bony prominence. A flexible faceplate that can adjust to the bony hump is another possibility, as is a custom-made faceplate. If no reusable appliance can be made to fit securely, then a disposable appliance is probably the best solution.

When the stoma is located in an incision or near a retention suture, the problem is reversed. Rather than compensate for a bony lump, we

now must fill in a depression. The best technique is to apply a small amount of skin barrier paste at the edge of the incision or over the edge of the retention sutures (Fig. 2-38), thus smoothing over the channel that undermines the faceplate seal. One can then apply surgical cement over the paste and skin area, cover the whole with a pliable skin barrier, and use a flexible disposable pouch.

A large peristomal hernia resulting in routine protuberance of the area can best be fitted with a disposable appliance, either two-piece (wafer and snap-on pouch) or one-piece with a skin barrier. Sometimes this problem can be managed with a reusable appliance, but it must have a flexible faceplate.

When the stoma is retracted or located in a skin fold, the faceplate convexity must match the degree of retraction to give a close fit at the base of the stoma. If the convexity is not deep enough, a gap exists between the plate and the skin, allowing urine to undermine the adhesive. If the convexity of the plate is too deep, the plate is not stable and rocks on the abdomen. If the skin fold is on both sides of the stoma, a custom-made elliptical convex faceplate may work better than a round faceplate.

An elliptical or odd-shaped stoma requires custom fitting. One can custom-cut a reusable plastic faceplate, order a custom-made appliance from a manufacturer, or use a disposable pouch and custom cut each adhesive.

Hyperplasia around a stoma is usually a reaction to urine (Fig. 2-39). To treat it, one should select a faceplate that fits close to the

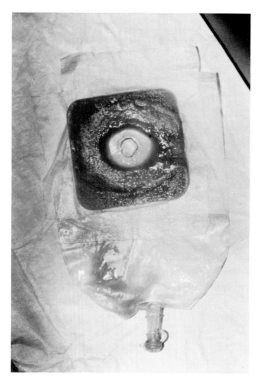

**Figure 2-40.** A skin barrier has been removed from a urinary stoma. The skin indicates that the barrier melted and absorbed urine on its outer edges, which left the skin in constant contact with urine.

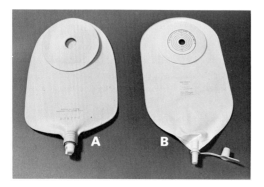

**Figure 2-41.** Two examples of one-piece presized urinary pouches: (*A*) Perma-Type; (*B*) Nu Hope.

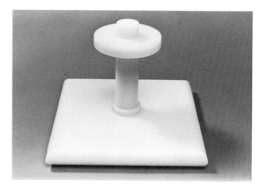

**Figure 2-42.** A device called "The Third Hand," to assist a patient assemble and apply a two-piece reusable appliance.

stoma, providing firm support and preventing urine from contacting the skin. Each time the pouch is changed, the hyperplasia can be softened by an application of full-strength vinegar to the skin. The skin gradually softens and is pushed back from the stoma by the faceplate. A skin barrier is detrimental here, because the barrier absorbs urine, leaving the skin constantly wet (Fig. 2-40).

Dexterity problems are fairly common in elderly cancer patients. Careful appliance selection, however, can make it possible for these patients to be independent. One option is to select a one-piece presized appliance that requires no cutting or assembly (Fig. 2-41). If it is disposable, all the patient must do is remove the adhesive backing. If it is reusable, the patient can either paint surgical cement on the skin and the plate or can apply a precut double-faced adhesive to the plate. If all of these procedures are too difficult, the patient may be able to wear a nonadhesive urinary appliance that requires minimal assembly and is applied simply by attaching a belt.

For some patients, the solution is an ingenious device called "The Third Hand" (Fig. 2-42). This device allows the patient to assemble the faceplate and tape on the "Third Hand" stand. The stand is a hollow tubular device calibrated to the size of the stoma. After the plate and adhesive are in place, the patient places the tube and plate over the stoma. The urine collects in the hollow tube while the patient dries his skin. He then slips the faceplate down the stand into position around the stoma and presses the adhesive and tape onto the skin.

## Long-term Follow-up

When a patient returns to the clinic after his first period at home, he has had time to practice caring for the stoma, learning what works well and what seems difficult. At this time we reevaluate the patient by assessing the stoma, the appliance, and the patient's home care. We look at the patient's needs for further learning, the methods of care, the fit of the appliance, the condition of the skin, the character and size of the stoma, the patient's involvement in routine activities (social, work, and sexual), and the patient's emotional response to living with an ostomy. Further teaching may be appropriate at this time.

We believe that every patient should be carefully examined on each successive follow-up visit. The follow-up visit offers an opportunity to identify and begin resolving any problems that have developed. These can be primarily physical or primarily emotional, but are frequently interrelated; both require attention. The gentleman who has had a conduit for ten years may verbally profess no problems, yet an examination can reveal a poorly fitting outdated appliance and hyperplasia. Another patient may appear to have no physical problems, but when she is questioned she admits that she sleeps with a plastic sheet on her bed and refuses to visit her in-laws for fear of leakage at night. These problems are solvable and should not go unattended.

## CONCLUSION

A urinary diversion performed in a patient with cancer is a serious matter. The choice of surgical technique and of stoma site require careful appraisal. The consequences affect daily personal care and are permanent. In addition, the behavior of the members of the health care team who participate in the patient's care can significantly affect his or her physical and emotional recovery. The goal of the urinary diversion, combined with cancer therapy, is full recovery. This includes rehabilitation of the patient—a return to his former life-style—and is attainable.

## APPENDIX 2-1

## Manufacturers of Disposable and Reusable Appliances

*Disposable*

1. Conva Tec
   A Squibb Company
   P. O. Box 4000, 1
   Princeton, NJ 08540
2. Coloplast, Inc.
   6206 Benjamin Road
   Tampa, FL 33614
3. Dansac
   2920 Wolff Street
   P. O. Box 4089
   Racine, WI 53404
4. Hollister, Inc.
   2000 Hollister Drive
   Libertyville, IL 60048
5. Mason Laboratories, Inc.
   Box 334
   Horsham, PA 19044

*Reusable*

1. Atlantic Surgical Co., Inc.
   1834 Lansdowne Avenue
   Merrick, NY 11566
2. Perma-Type Co., Inc.
   P. O. 448
   Farmington, CT 06032
3. Tarbot Co.
   1185 Jefferson Boulevard
   Warwick, RI 02886-2298
4. Vance
   VPI
   1100 West Morgan Street
   P. O. Box 266
   Spencer, IN 47460

*Disposable and Reusable*

1. Bard Home Heath Division
   C. R. Bard, Inc.
   Berkeley Heights, NJ 07922
2. Gricks
   202-11 Jamaica Avenue
   Hollis, NY 11423
3. John F. Greer Company
   530 E. 12th Street
   Oakland, CA 94606

4. Marlen
5150 Richmond Rd.
Bedford, OH 44146
5. Nu Hope
P. O. Box 39348
Los Angeles, CA 90039
6. United
Division of Howmedica, Inc.
Largo, FL 33540

## APPENDIX 2-2

### Helpful Hints for the Patient with a Urinary Diversion

1. Drink six to eight glasses of liquid daily.
2. Keep the appliance and equipment clean.
3. Change the appliance every five to seven days.
4. Vitamin C tablets (500 mg three times a day) may help reduce urine alkalinity and odor.
5. Change your appliance in the morning before you have had anything to drink or in the evening before the dinner meal. Urinary output is lower at these times.
6. You may bathe or shower with the appliance either on or off. Water does not hurt the stoma or run into the opening.
7. Resume your normal recreational activities such as swimming, skiing, golf, bowling. If you have questions, check with your surgeon.

8. At night, connect your appliance to a urinary bedside drainage bag or put the tubing into a disposable container such as a plastic milk or Clorox bottle. Clean the tubing and container with vinegar or Clorox. According to your preference and sleep positions, the night-drain tubing can go off the side of the bed, down to the foot of the bed, or downwards and then under the thigh toward the side of the bed. The latter position keeps the tube from twisting and allows it to move with your leg as you turn from side to side.
9. Keep an extra adhesive and appliance with you for emergency needs. Women can carry extras in a cosmetic kit and men can use a shaving kit.
10. Take along a change of appliance when you visit your physician or ET nurse, as they will probably want to examine your stoma and skin.
11. If you are admitted to a hospital, take your own ostomy supplies. Hospitals may not have your particular appliance on hand.
12. When traveling, keep some of your ostomy supplies with you in case your luggage is lost.
13. Keep your equipment clean. Wash reusable equipment with warm, soapy water. A capful of vinegar or commercial mouthwash added to the water is helpful as a deodorant for the pouch.

## REFERENCES

1. Albertson PC, Albertson PS: Evaluation of a new nonadhesive urine collection device for patients with ileal conduits. J Urol 131:454–455, 1984
2. Anderson HV, Hodges CV, Behnam AM, Ocker JM Jr: Transureters-ureterostomy (contralateral uretero-ureterostomy): Experimental and clinical experiences. J Urol 83:593–601, 1960
3. Assadnia A, Lee CN, Petre JH, Lyons RC: Two cases of stone formation in ileal conduits after using staple gun for closure of proximal end of isolated loop. J Urol 108:553, 1972
4. Beaugie JM: Fistula between external iliac artery and ileal conduit. Br J Urol 43:450–452, 1973
5. Bergman SM, Sears HF, Javadpour N: Compli-

cation with mechanical stapling device in creation of ileoconduit. Urology 12:71–73, 1978
6. Bishop RF, Smith ED, Gracey M: Bacterial flora of urine from ileal conduit. J Urol 105:452–455, 1971
7. Bisson JM, Vinson RK, Leadbetter GW: Urolithiasis from stapler anastomosis. Am J Surg 137:280–282, 1979
8. Bloom DA, Lieskovsky G, Rainwater G, Skinner DG: The Turnbull loop stoma. J Urol 129:715–718, 1983
9. Bracken RB, McDonald M, Johnson DE: Complications of single-stage radical cystectomy and ileal conduit. Urology 17:141–146, 1981
10. Bricker EM: Bladder substitution after pelvic evisceration. Surg Clin North Am 30:1511–1521, 1950

11. Bricker EM: The evolution of the ileal segment bladder substitution operation. Am J Surg 135:834–841, 1978

12. Broadwell DC, Appleby CH, Bates MA, Jackson BS: Principles and techniques of pouching, in Broadwell DC, Jackson BS (Eds): Principles of Ostomy Care. St. Louis, C. V. Mosby, 1982, pp 565–643

13. Bruce Medical Supply Fall 1985 Buyers Guide, Waltham, Mass.

14. Bystrom J: Early and late complications of ileal conduit urinary diversion. Scand J Urol Nephrol 12:233–237, 1978

15. Caponegro PJ, Leadbetter GW Jr: Acute ureteral obstruction secondary to mucoid impaction in supravesical diversion: Treatment with N-acetylcysteine. Urology 3:486–487, 1974

16. Chiang MS, Minton JP, Clausen K, et al: Carcinoma in a colon conduit urinary diversion. J Urol 127:1185–1187, 1982

17. Clark SS: Electrolyte disturbance associated with jejunal conduit. J Urol 112:42–47, 1974

18. Clark SS: High urinary diversion by retroperitoneal jejunal conduit: Technique and rationale. Rev Surg 30:1–5, 1973

19. Click C: Care of the patient with a urinary diversion. Cancer Bull 33:15–18, 1981

20. Cohen SM, Persky L: A ten-year experience with ureteroileostomy. Arch Surg 95:278–283, 1967

21. Daughtry JD, Susan LP, Stewart BH, Straffon RA: Ileal conduit and cystectomy: A 10-year retrospective study of ileal conduits performed in conjunction with cystectomy and with a minimum 5-year followup. J Urol 118:556–557, 1977

22. David FRD: A new surgical procedure for revision of ileal conduit stoma in children. J Urol 115:188–190, 1976

23. DeVries JK: Permanent diversion of the urinary stream. J Urol 73:217–225, 1955

24. Dretler SP: The pathogenesis of urinary tract calculi occurring after ileal conduit diversion: I. Clinical study. II. Conduit study. III. Prevention. J Urol 109:204–209, 1973

25. Dunn M, Roberts JBM, Smith PJB, Slade N: The long-term results of ileal conduit urinary diversion in children. Br J Urol 51:458–461, 1979

26. Eckhauser FE, Sonda LP, Strodel WE, et al: Parastomal ileal conduit hemorrhage and portal hypertension. Ann Surg 192:620–624, 1980

27. Eckstein HB: Ureteral diversion, in Glenn JF (Ed): Urologic Surgery (3rd ed). Philadelphia, J. B. Lippincott, 1983, pp 491–499

28. Elder DD, Moisey CU, Rees RWM: A long-term follow-up of the colonic conduit operation in children. Br J Urol 51:462–465, 1979

29. Elliot TE, Albertazzi VJ, Danto LA: Stenosis after stapler anastomosis. Am J Surg 133:750–751, 1977

30. Esho J, Ireland G, Blackard C, Cass A: Late stenosis of bowel segment of ileac conduit (pipestem loop). Urology 3:30–33, 1974

31. Firlit RS, Firlit CF, Canning J: Exsanguinating hemorrhage from urinary ileal conduit in patient with portal hypertension. Urology 12:710–711, 1978

32. Fowler JW, Hart AJL, Duncan W: The effects of radiotherapy on the integrity of the ureteroileal segment following cystectomy. Br J Urol 54:126–129, 1982

33. Gigon C: Mémoire sur l'ischurie urétérique et sur l'urétérotomie ou taille de l'urétere. Union Med Paris 10:81, 1856

34. Gluck T, Zeller A: Über extirpation der Harnblase und Prostata. Arch Klin Chir 26:916–924, 1881

35. Golimbu M, Morales M: Jejunal conduits: Technique and complications. J Urol 113:787–795, 1975

36. Gonzales ET Jr, Baum NH, Friedman A, Carlton CE: Sigmoid conduit: Review and description of technique. Urology 10:579–581, 1977

37. Gregory JG, Gursahani M, Schoenberg HW: Five-year radiographic review of ileal conduits. J Urol 112:327–331, 1974

38. Grimes JH: Stone disease in urinary diversion. South Med J 68:1494–1496, 1975

39. Halverstadt DB, Fraley EE: Perforation of ileal segment by calculi formed on nonabsorbable suture material: Unusual complications of ileal conduit diversion. J Urol 102:188–190, 1969

40. Hanafy HM: Mid-ureteral leakage: An unusual complication of ileal conduit. J Urol 118:679, 1977

41. Hardy BE, Lebowitz RL, Baez A, Colodny AH: Strictures of the ileal loop. J Urol 117:358–361, 1977

42. Hendry WF: Urinary diversion in the adult, in Todd IP (Ed): Intestinal Stomas. London, Heinemann, 1982, pp 113–124

43. Heney NM, Dretler SP, Hensle TW, Kerr WS Jr: Autosuturing device in intestinal urinary conduits. Urology 12:650–653, 1978

44. Hensle TW, Bredin HC, Dretler SP: Diagnosis and treatment of a urinary leak after ureteroileal conduit for diversion. J Urol 116:29–31, 1975

45. Higgins RB: Bilateral transperitoneal umbilical ureterostomy. J Urol 921:289–294, 1964

46. Hill JT, Ransley PG: The colonic conduit: A better method of urinary diversion? Br J Urol 55:629–631, 1983

47. Hindmarsh JR: Common iliac-ileal conduit fistula. Br J Urol 49:508, 1977

48. Hinman F, Smith A: Total cystectomy for cancer: A critical review. Surgery 6:851–881, 1939

49. Hinman F, Weyrauch HM Jr: A critical study of the different principles of surgery which have been used in uretero-intestinal implantation. Trans Am Assoc Genitourin Surg 29:15–156, 1936

50. Holden S, Whitmore WF Jr: Ureter diversion, in Bergman H (Ed): The Ureter (2nd ed). New York, Springer-Verlag, 1981, pp 717–754

51. Hopkins TB, Trento A: Parastomal ileal loop hernia repair with Marlex mesh. J Urol 128:811–812, 1982

52. Jaffe BM, Bricker EM, Butcher HR Jr: Surgical complications of ileal segment urinary diversion. Ann Surg 167:367–376, 1968

53. Jeter K: Better care for the ostomy patient. Am Surg 39:124–126, 1973

54. Jeter KF: Evaluating the merits of a new nonadhesive urostomy appliance. Am Urol Assoc Allied J 4:4–7, 1983

55. Jeter KF: The flush versus the protruding urinary stoma. J Urol 116:424–427, 1976

56. Johnson DE, Fuerst DE: Use of autosuture for construction of ileal conduit. J Urol 109:821–823, 1973

57. Johnson DE, Lamy SM: Complications of a single stage radical cystectomy and ileal conduit diversion: Review of 214 cases. J Urol 117:171–173, 1977

58. Johnson DE, Jackson L, Guinn GA: Ileal conduit diversion for carcinoma of the bladder. South Med J 63:1115–1118, 1970

59. Johnson JH, Rickman PP: Complications following ureteroileostomy in childhood and the use of cutaneous ureterostomy in advanced lesions. Br J Urol 30:437–449, 1958

60. Kaplan AL, Hulme GW, Laskowski T, Calhoun CA: The sigmoid conduit as a means of urinary diversion. South Med J 60:688–691, 1967

61. Karamcheti A, O'Donnell WF, Hakala TR, et al: Autosuture ileal conduit construction: Experience in 110 cases. J Urol 120:545–548, 1978

62. Kaufman JJ, Jeter KF: "O" ring urinary ostomy appliance. Urology 23:180–182, 1984

63. Kinn AC, Johansson B: Volvulus of an ileal conduit as a lethal complication of urinary diversion: Report of one case. Scand J Urol Nephrol 16:77–78, 1982

64. Kochevar J: Adenocarcinoid tumor, goblet cell type, arising in a ureteroileal conduit: A case report. J Urol 131:957–959, 1984

65. Lapides J: Butterfly cutaneous ureterostomy. J Urol 88:735–739, 1962

66. Laurenze, 1888. Cited by Papin E: Chirurgie du Rein, vol 3. Paris, Doin, 1928

67. Leadbetter WF, Clarke BG: Five year experience with uretero-enterostomy by the combined technique. J Urol 73:67–82, 1954

68. Le Dentu A: Greffe de l'uretere entre les levres d'une incision du flanc chez une femme atteinte d'anurie absolu. Cong Franc Urol 4:533, 1890

69. Lloyd FA, Cattrell TLC, Cross RR, Calens J: High cutaneous ureterostomy. J Urol 88:740–745, 1962

70. Lo RK, Johnson DE, Smith DB: Massive bleeding from an ileal conduit caput medusae. J Urol 131:114–115, 1984

71. Lynne CM, Politano VA, Cohen RL: Parastomal hernia causing anuria. Urology 4:603–604, 1974

72. Manson W, Collen S, Forsberg L, et al: Renal function after urinary diversion: A study of continent caecal reservoir ileal conduit and colonic conduit. Scand J Urol Nephrol 18:307–315, 1984

73. Manson W, Ekelund AL, Sundin T: Severe bleeding from urinary conduits: A case report. Scand J Urol Nephrol 16:295–298, 1982

74. Marshall FF, Leadbetter WF, Dretler SP: Ileal conduit parastomal hernias. J Urol 114:40–42, 1975

75. McEwan AB, Clark P: The stoma of the ileal conduit. Br J Urol 45:600–605, 1973

76. McLaughlin TC: Crohn's disease developing in an ileal conduit. J Urol 125:420–421, 1981

77. Mersheimer WL, Kolarsick AJ, Kammandel H: Implantation of ureters into completely isolated loops of small intestine. Proc Soc Exp Biol Med 76:170–171, 1951

78. Mersheimer WL, Kolarsick AJ, Kammandel H: Method for construction of artificial urinary bladder by implantation of ureters into completely or partially excluded segments of small intestine. Bull NY Med Coll 13:71–77, 1950

79. Mitchell ME, Yoder IC, Daly PJ, Althausen A: Ileal loop stenosis: A late complication of urinary diversion. J Urol 118:957–961, 1977

80. Mogg R: Some observations on urinary diversion. Ann R Coll Surg Engl 46:251–266, 1970

81. Mogg RA: The treatment of urinary incontinence using the colonic conduit. Trans Am Assoc Genitourin Surg 58:90–101, 1966

82. Mogg RA, Syme RRA: The results of urinary diversion using the colonic conduit. Br J Urol 41:434–447, 1969

83. Morales P, Golimbu M: Colonic urinary diversion: 10 years of experience. J Urol 113:302–307, 1975

84. Morales PA, Whitehead ED: Commentary on cutaneous ureterostomy, in Whitehead ED (Ed): Current Operative Urology. New York, Harper and Row, 1957, pp 451–458

85. Morales PA, Whitehead ED: High jejunal conduit for supravesical urinary diversion. Urology 1:426–431, 1973

86. Myers RP, Rife CC, Barrett DM: Experience with the bowel stapler for ileal conduit urinary diversion. J Urol 54:491–493, 1982

87. Nance FC: New techniques of gastrointestinal anastomosis with the EEA stapler. Am Surg 189:587–699, 1979

88. Nichols WK, Krause AH, Donegan WL: Urinary fistulas after ureteral diversion. Am J Surg 124:311–316, 1972

89. Nieh PT, Parkhurst EC: Successful management of ileal conduit-enteric fistula: The case against loopograms. J Urol 118:112–113, 1977

90. Orr JW, Shingleton HM, Hatch KD, et al: Urinary diversion in patients undergoing pelvic exenteration. Am J Obstet Gynecol 142:883–889, 1982

91. Palmer JM: Island pedicle graft in stomal stenosis: A new technique. J Urol 130:453–455, 1983

92. Perlmutter AD: Spiral advancement skin flap for stomal revision. J Urol 114:131–132, 1975

93. Peterson NE: Adenoma of ileal urinary conduit. J Urol 131:1171–1172, 1984

94. Pitts WR Jr: Crohn's disease developing in ileal conduit (Letter to editor). J Urol 127:554, 1982

95. Poor P, Kursh ED, Persky L: The add-on ileal loop. J Urol 114:281–284, 1975

96. Preissig RS, Barry WF Jr, Lester RG: The increased incidence of carcinoma of the colon following ureterosigmoidostomy. Am J Roentgenol 121:806–810, 1974

97. Redman JF: A technique for correction of ileocutaneous stomal stenosis. J Urol 119:333–334, 1978

98. Rodriguez DB: Management of urinary stomas, in Johnson DE, Boileau MA (Eds): Genitourinary Tumors: Fundamental Principles and Surgical Techniques. New York, Grune & Stratton, 1982, pp 519–529

99. Rodriguez DB: Stoma care. Clin Gastroenterol 2:318–326, 1982

100. Rosen RJ, McLean GK, Freiman DB, et al: Obstructed ureteroileal conduits: Antegrade catheter drainage. AJR 135:1201–1204, 1980

101. Seiffert L: Die 'Darm Siphon-Blase.' Arch Klin Chir 183:569, 1935

102. Shortland JR, Spencer RC, Williams JL: Pseudomembranous colitis associated with changes in an ileal conduit. J Clin Pathol 36:1184–1187, 1983

103. Shousha S, Scott J, Polak J: Ileal loop carcinoma after cystectomy for bladder exstrophy. Br Med J 2:397–398, 1978

104. Smith AD, Lange PH, Miller RP, Reinke DB: Percutaneous dilatation of ureteroileal strictures and insertion of Gibbons ureteral stents. Urology 13:24–26, 1979

105. Smith DB: Reusable appliances. J Enterostom Ther 11(2):71–73, 1984

106. Spence B, Stewart W, Cass AS: Use of a double-lumen catheter to determine bacteriuria in intestinal loop diversions in children. J Urol 108:800–801, 1972

107. Straffen RA, Kyle H, Corvalon J: Techniques of cutaneous ureterostomy and results in 51 patients. J Urol 103:138–146, 1970

108. Sullivan JW, Grabstald H, Whitmore WF Jr: Complications of ureteroileal conduit with radical cystectomy: Review of 336 cases. J Urol 124:797–801, 1980

109. Swan RW, Rutledge F: Urinary conduit in pelvic cancer patients: A report of 16 years' experience. Am J Obstet Gynecol 119:6–13, 1974

110. Symmonds RE, Gibbs CP: Urinary diversion by way of sigmoid conduit. Surg Gynecol Obstet 131:687–693, 1970

111. Thompson IM, Ross GR Jr: Experiences with a new technique for supravesical diversion. J Urol 90:691–695, 1963

112. Tomera KM, Unni KK, Utz DC: Adenomatous polyp in ileal conduit. J Urol 128:1025–1026, 1982

113. Urdonita LF, Duffell D, Creeney CD, Aust JB: Late development of primary carcinoma of the colon following ureterosigmoidostomy: Report of three cases and literature review. Ann Surg 164:503–513, 1966

114. Walsh A: Urinary diversion in malignant disease, in Ashken MH (Ed): Urinary Diversion. New York, Springer-Verlag, 1982, pp 75–100

115. Wassiljew MA: Über Totalextirpation der Harnblase bei bösartiger Neubildung. Russki Khir Arkh 4:31, 1895

116. Winter CC: Cutaneous omento-ureterostomy: Clinical application. J Urol 107:233–238, 1972

117. Wood RY: Catheterizing the patient with an ileal conduit stoma. Am J Nurs 76:1592–1595, 1976

118. Wright NE: Caput medusae in portal hypertension. J Enterostom Ther 8(2):17–20, 1981

119. Zaayer: Discussion. Intra-abdominale Plastieken. Ned Tijdschr Geneeskd 65:836, 1911

120. Zink M: Double-lumen versus single-lumen catheterization of ileal/colon conduits. J Enterostom Ther 11(2):190–195, 1984

David M. Gershenson
Dorothy B. Smith

# 3

# Enteric Diversions

Enteric diversions, i.e., colostomies and ileostomies, have a strange internal dichotomy. They have the potential of either saving a life or destroying a life. They may even, at the same time, do both.

There are always two aspects of a bowel diversion: the external or physical and the internal or emotional. Caring for or teaching the patient with an intestinal stoma can never be limited to only one of these aspects. Attention to both is required to sustain the physical and the emotional life of the patient.

However, in this chapter we focus intentionally on the mechanics of enteric diversions: the when, the why, and the how to. Satisfactorily managing these mechanics is the prerequisite to helping the patient adjust emotionally to a colostomy or an ileostomy. If the ostomy is constructed in a manner that does not permit appliance security or if the patient is not taught how to care for the ostomy, acceptance and rehabilitation are unattainable goals. The physical life saved may become an emotional life destroyed.

## COLOSTOMY

### Historical Development

The first reports of an opening into the colon date back to biblical times: in the third book of Judges, Eglon, the King of Moab, was stabbed by Ehud and died from a bowel perforation.[6,25] Cheselden, a British surgeon, reported in 1784 of a patient of his who spontaneously developed a "preternatural" connection between her bowel and her skin because of an obstructing umbilical hernia.[4] The bowel erupted through the umbilicus as a fistula. Cheselden trimmed the sloughing bowel and the patient survived several years, passing stool through her abdominal opening. Historically, it was a rare incident when a patient with a bowel obstruction or perforation did not die.

Alexis Littre, a French surgeon, first suggested a colostomy, although he did not actually perform one.[6,25] While performing a postmortem examination on a six-day-old baby boy who had died with an imperforate anus, he suggested that the upper end of the bowel could have been brought out of the abdominal cavity and sewn to the skin to let gas and feces escape. The first colostomy performed was by Pillare of Rouen, France, in 1776,[6,7,25] when he operated on a man for bowel obstruction. Although the operation was considered a surgical success, the patient died, not from the surgery, but from mercury that had been placed in his bowel before surgery to work its way through the obstruction. Duret, a French surgeon, read of Alexis Littre's suggestion and, in 1793, constructed a sigmoid colostomy in a three-day-old infant with an imperforate anus.[6] The patient lived for 45 years. Over a seven-year period beginning in 1826, Lisfranc operated on nine patients who had rectal carcinomas.[9] He excised the distal portion of the rectum, including the sphincter, and sutured the proximal end of the bowel to the skin of the perineum, creating a perineal colostomy.

Although successful colostomy operations were reported occasionally, most patients died due to contamination of the peritoneal cavity from feces and the subsequent peritonitis.[6] In an effort to reduce peritoneal contamination, Amussat performed a lumbar colostomy in 1839.[6,14] The operation was successful, and thereafter became a popular way of relieving colonic obstruction in the nineteenth century. However, the stoma's position made it impossible for the patient to see and difficult to fit with an appliance; the stoma also tended to stricture. In 1884, when Czerny was removing the rectum of a patient with rectal carcinoma and found he was unable to bring the amputated bowel to the lumbar region, he brought it out through the abdominal wall.[9] This technique was further developed by Volkmann (1887), Gaudier (1896), and Kraske (1900).[9]

Early in the twentieth century, Miles (1908) described an abdominoperineal resection and creation of an abdominal stoma, and Hartmann (1921) published his procedure for removing tumors in the upper rectum, leaving a rectal pouch and an abdominal stoma.[9] In 1950 two British surgeons, Goligher and Patey, independently suggested two additional procedures: bringing the colostomy through an extraperitoneal tunnel to prevent internal herniation of the small intestine, and opening the intestinal loop during surgery and sewing it to the skin to prevent stoma stricture.[11]

### Indications

Colostomies, either temporary or permanent, are no longer relegated to emergencies resulting from obstruction, perforation, or trauma. Improvements in surgical techniques, in postoperative nursing care, and in available appliances have made colostomy surgery an acceptable treatment in a variety of situations.

In a patient with cancer, indications for a colostomy are varied. Any type of pelvic mass that has the potential of causing bowel obstruction or perforation may necessitate a colostomy.[23] Specific indications include: (1) removal of the entire rectum and distal colon for cancer of the rectum, cervix, bladder, or prostate; (2)

decompression of a bowel partially or completely obstructed by a lesion believed to be resectable, which later can be irradiated or surgically removed; (3) protection of a bowel anastomosis lower in the colon; (4) diversion of the fecal stream above a colonic fistula— rectovaginal, rectovesical, or enterocutaneous; (5) diversion of the fecal stream above an area of the colon that has been inflamed or injured by, for example, perforation, abscess formation, or radiation injury; (6) decompression of a bowel partially or completely obstructed by stenosis or stricture from radiation changes; and (7) diversion of the fecal stream above an unresectable obstructing lesion.

### Preoperative Preparation

An important part of the planned care for patients who are to have a colostomy takes place before surgery (see Chapter 1). Patients are admitted to the hospital a few days before the date surgery is scheduled to follow an appropriately restricted diet and to undergo mechanical and antibiotic bowel preparation. Of course this preparation is impossible if the patient has a colonic obstruction or perforation; in this instance, a surgical emergency exists.

During the preoperative period, the physician, nurse, social worker, dietician, and enterostomal therapist counsel the patient. They explain the indications for and possible complications of the procedure, describe the procedure itself, and discuss postoperative management of the stoma, possible changes in diet, and prospects for returning to normal activities. These members of the health care team answer questions from patient and family and attempt to alleviate concerns about the effects of the stoma on the patient's daily life.

The site of the stoma should be selected prior to surgery. If the surgery is to be an end sigmoid colostomy for rectal carcinoma, one stoma site may be selected on the left according to the principles in Chapter 1. If, however, surgery is for an ovarian malignancy that may involve multiple areas of bowel obstruction or tumor implants in the mesentery, the surgeon may be uncertain about which type of colostomy to perform, i.e., a right or left transverse or a descending colostomy. In such situations more than one site should be selected and marked—a left and right transverse site and a descending site. After the surgical incision has been made is too late to determine a secondary stoma site. Marking multiple stoma sites on patients with several areas of either small or large bowel obstruction also gives the surgeon a proper site in which to locate mucous fistulas if they are needed.

Selecting a stoma site may be difficult on patients with intestinal obstruction or large abdominal masses because of the resulting distorted abdomen. The bony prominences and surgical scars can be located, but natural abdominal creases become obliterated by the distention. Questioning the patient about his beltline or natural abdominal crease may help.

When the physician and nurse mark multiple stoma sites, they should be certain to explain why several sites are selected and assure the patient that the multiple marks do not necessarily mean multiple stomas.

## Colostomy Construction

Although colostomies may be classified according to the associated urgency (emergency or elective), the expected duration (permanent or temporary), the site (ascending, transverse, descending, or sigmoid), or the purpose (decompression of an obstruction; diversion of the fecal stream because of a fistula, a perforation, or a precarious anastomosis; or tumor removal), for purposes of this chapter we will discuss the types of colostomy according to their methods of construction. The three major types are: (1) the loop colostomy, (2) the end colostomy, and (3) the Turnbull or decompression colostomy.

Physiologically, the right and left portions of the colon differ markedly. The major function of the right colon is water absorption. The ascending and transverse portions of the colon possess peristaltic activity. Conversely, the left colon functions as a reservoir through which stool is propelled by mass action. The stool in a transverse colostomy is therefore more liquid than the solid stool of the descending or sigmoid colostomy. A patient with a transverse colostomy usually must wear an appliance constantly, but the patient with a descending colostomy may control output nicely with regular irrigations.

### The Loop Colostomy

In a patient with cancer, the loop colostomy is usually employed for one of the following purposes: (1) to relieve acute obstruction from tumor, either primary or metastatic, or from irradiation stricture; (2) to protect a distal anastomosis; or (3) as a diverting procedure to avoid a distal irradiation proctitis, perforation, or fistula. In the latter situation, many surgeons prefer a completely separated or double-barrel end colostomy. The decision between a transverse or descending colostomy is determined by many factors, including the patient's age, weight, and general medical condition, the location of the problem, and the associated urgency. All things being equal, a descending colostomy is preferable since its stool is more solid and more easily controlled with irrigation. On the other hand, the descending colon mesentery is much less mobile, and more operative time is required to mobilize it. Therefore, a descending loop colostomy may not be feasible in an obese patient or a patient who is medically unstable. In addition, tumor or radiation fibrosis may make adequate mobilization impossible.

One may employ either a transverse incision two to three fingerbreadths above the umbilicus over the right or left rectus muscles (for a right or left transverse loop colostomy) or a midline incision (for a descending or sigmoid loop colostomy). A word of caution about choosing an incision is indicated: if the surgeon is performing a transverse loop colostomy in a patient with extensive intraabdominal carcinomatosis, a small transverse incision may not allow adequate enough exposure to mobilize a portion of transverse colon.

After making the incision, the surgeon chooses the segment of bowel with which to construct the colostomy. If it is transverse colon, the surgeon may need to dissect the omentum away from the portion selected; if it is descending colon, he may need to mobilize the mesentery by incising the peritoneum in the left paracolic gutter or by dissecting the splenic flexure from its surrounding attachments. If the latter technique is necessary, the surgeon should be careful not to injure the spleen. Once the mesentery and segment of colon are adequately mobilized, a Penrose drain is placed through an avascular location where the bowel wall is attached to the mesentery (Fig. 3-1). The drain is used for gentle traction to deliver the colon through the incision.

When the operation is performed through a midline incision, the surgeon must construct a separate stoma. In this situation, an assistant

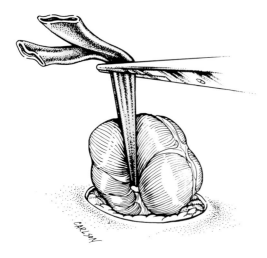

**Figure 3-1.** A Penrose drain is placed through an avascular area in the mesentery and used for gentle traction.

first grasps the fascia with a Kocher clamp and the skin with an Allis clamp and draws these tissues medially to align the layers of the abdominal wall, thereby avoiding a scissoring effect. At the same time, the surgeon grasps the previously marked stoma site with a Kocher clamp and makes a circumferential incision 2–3 cm in diameter. He then incises vertically the underlying subcutaneous tissue and fascia, exposing the rectus abdominis muscle. After bluntly separating the muscle with a clamp, he makes an opening in the peritoneum. The aperture should admit two fingers easily. The drain around the colon is then passed through the stoma aperture, and the colon is brought through.

Once the colon has been delivered through the chosen incision, the surgeon slips a bridge just under the drain, removes the drain, and attaches the bridge to the skin with 3-0 nylon sutures (Fig. 3-2). As an alternative technique,

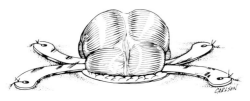

**Figure 3-2.** A colostomy bridge is sutured to the skin with 3-0 nylon sutures.

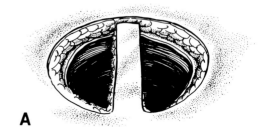

**A**

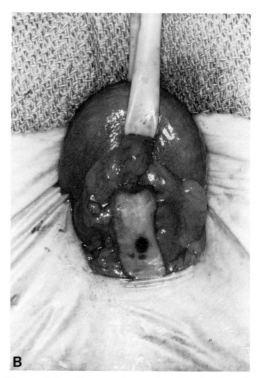

**B**

**Figure 3-3.** Construction of a skin bridge. **A,** schema; **B,** operative view.

instead of using a plastic bridge, the surgeon can construct a skin bridge (Fig. 3-3).

If a separate stoma aperture has been made, the midline incision is now closed. The bowel is then opened, by making either a longitudinal incision along the taenia (Fig. 3-4*A*) or a U-shaped incision (Fig. 3-4*B*). The latter incision may allow the surgeon to evert the proximal limb further. To complete the stoma, the surgeon approximates the full thickness of the bowel wall to the skin with interrupted sutures of 3-0 plain or chromic catgut (Fig. 3-4*C*). If a

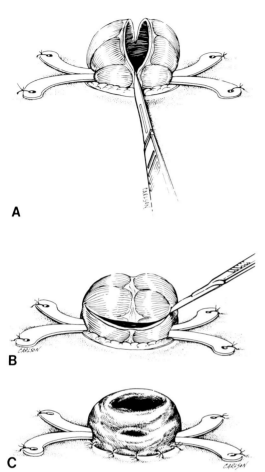

**A**

**B**

**C**

**Figure 3-4.** Maturing the stoma. The physician may choose to open the colon with either **A**, a longitudinal incision along the taenia, or **B**, a U-shaped incision. **C**, the colon wall is approximated to the skin with interrupted sutures of 3-0 plain catgut.

plastic bridge has been used, it is removed seven to ten days postoperatively.

### The End Colostomy

The most common use of the end colostomy in patients who have cancer is in conjunction with an abdominoperineal resection for carcinoma of the rectum. An end sigmoid or descending colostomy may also be performed without a rectal resection, in which case the distal end of bowel is brought to the surface as a mucous fistula, or in association with partial resection of the distal colon, in which case the distal end of bowel is oversewn and returned to the peritoneal

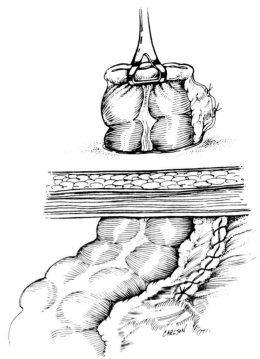

**Figure 3-5.** Constructing an end colostomy. The transected end of the colon is delivered through the stomal aperture. Note that the mesentery has been sutured to the lateral peritoneum to prevent future internal hernia. (The stoma is completed by approximating the bowel wall to the skin with interrupted sutures of 3-0 plain catgut.)

cavity (Hartmann operation). Indications for these latter procedures include a distal fistula and a perforation.

Most procedures that employ an end colostomy begin with a midline incision. Once the initial portion of the surgery is completed (e.g., abdominoperineal resection for cancer of the rectum or partial resection of the rectosigmoid for radiation-induced injury, perforation, or tumor), the stoma aperture is constructed just as described above for a loop colostomy. If necessary, the mesentery of the colon is mobilized by incising the peritoneum in the left paracolic gutter or by freeing the attachments to the splenic flexure. The transected end of the colon is then gently delivered through the aperture with a clamp (Fig. 3-5). The colon should be free of tension, and the stomal aperture should be large enough to allow the mesentery adequate

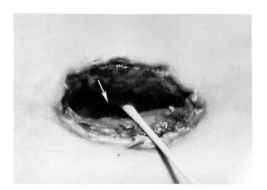

**Figure 3-6.** The bowel (arrow) has completely separated from the skin and has retracted into the abdominal wall.

room yet small enough to help prevent future problems with parastomal hernia. To prevent internal hernia formation, the surgeon obliterates the lateral paracolic gutter by suturing the bowel wall or the mesentery to the lateral peritoneum. Next, the midline incision is closed, after which the full thickness of bowel wall is approximated to the skin with interrupted sutures of 3-0 plain or chromic catgut.

If a mucous fistula is also brought to the surface, it requires a separate stoma aperture. If at all possible, one should avoid bringing the mucous fistula through the midline incision. It should also not be so close to the colostomy stoma that it interferes with proper fitting of the appliance.

### The Turnbull or Decompression Colostomy

When the colon is markedly dilated or when tumor fixation does not allow adequate colon mobilization, a decompression transverse colostomy may be indicated. One may use either a small transverse incision two to three fingerbreadths above the umbilicus or a midline incision plus a separate stomal incision.

Once the portion of transverse colon has been selected, it is mobilized as much as possible and delivered into the incision. If necessary, the dilated colon may be decompressed by puncturing it with a needle. The seromuscular layer of the colon is then sutured to the fascia with interrupted sutures of 3-0 silk. The colon wall is incised, and the open colon is grasped with Babcock clamps and elevated to the level of the

skin. The edges of the incised colon are then sutured to the surrounding skin with interrupted 3-0 plain or chromic catgut.

### Complications

Some of the surgical complications of a colostomy are structural and can be prevented. It is the surgeon's responsibility, through preoperative planning and intraoperative technique, to minimize postoperative complications.

#### Retraction

Stoma retraction is usually caused by either excessive tension on the stoma or inadequate blood supply to the stoma, resulting in ischemia and necrosis because of excessive devascularization of the bowel. Stoma retraction should be prevented by adequately mobilizing the bowel mesentery. Mesenteric fixation by tumor or by radiation fibrosis may make this especially difficult in some cancer patients. When patients are obese or have a thick wall of subcutaneous tissue, the need for bowel mobilization to get the stoma to the abdominal surface increases. If the tension is sufficient enough to pull the bowel away from the cutaneous suture line and back into the abdomen, surgical correction is necessary (Fig. 3-6). If the bowel stays intact at the fascia but retracts inward at the skin, the problem then becomes one of management: how to keep an appliance sealed (Fig. 3-7). If the retraction is such that an appliance will not stay in place, surgical revision is required. This procedure may simply consist of making a circumferential incision around the stoma, dissecting down to the fascial or peritoneal level, and advancing the bowel to construct a projecting nipple. More often, however, it requires repeat laparotomy, greater mobilization of the mesentery, and sometimes even relocation of the stoma.

#### Necrosis

A normal colostomy stoma is pink or reddish* and glistens. If its color darkens and it

---

\* An exception is a condition called melanosis coli, an increase of melanin in the mucosa. The result is a dull brownish appearance that can usually be seen throughout the colon. It is not related to blood supply but is associated with prolonged laxative abuse.

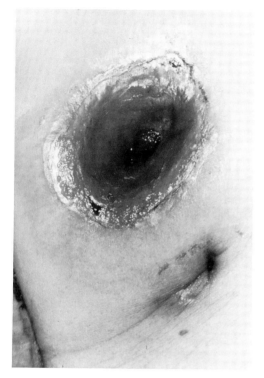

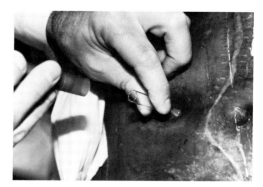

**Figure 3-8.** The physician has inserted a glass test tube into a stoma to observe the mucosa and determine if the necrotic process extends to the fascia level.

**Figure 3-7.** Severe stomal retraction has resulted in inadequate appliance seal and severe irritation.

shine a light through the tube, and look into the bowel to determine if the necrotic process extends to the fascia level. If it involves the intraperitoneal portion of the bowel, there is danger of perforation followed by peritonitis. If the ischemia is superficial, only the top of the bowel mucosa will slough. However, as the necrotic tissue is shed and the surrounding tissue heals, stomal stenosis or retraction may result.

*Stenosis*

Although new surgical techniques have reduced the occurrence of stomal stenosis, it is still a possible complication. It may result from a necrotic stoma that has healed or from peristomal infections or recurrent episodes of skin excoriation. Occasionally, stenosis occurs because the abdominal wall aperture was not made large enough. When the opening is not adequate, the result may be a stricture at either the fascial or skin level. Both the surgeon and the patient can prevent stenosis—the surgeon by employing careful surgical technique and avoiding those factors that predispose to stomal necrosis, and the patient by practicing meticulous stoma care. We used to believe that daily digital dilation of the colostomy would prevent stricture, but this is no longer considered necessary; some clinicians even believe it to be harmful, reasoning that the repeated dilation stretches and tears tissue, resulting in more scarring and further stenosis.

If the stenosis is severe enough to interfere

gradually turns black, necrosis should be suspected.

Stomal necrosis is usually caused by either devascularization or excessive tension. The marginal artery may have been injured, twisted, or occluded during surgery, or tension on the bowel may impede the blood supply. Necrosis can be prevented by adequately mobilizing the bowel mesentery and by avoiding excessive skeletonization of the bowel near the stoma.

If the surgeon spots an ischemic bowel at the time of the operation, he is well advised to redo the stoma at that time, rather than wait two or three days and have to perform a second laparotomy. An ischemic bowel is in danger of becoming gangrenous, retracting into the peritoneal cavity, and causing peritonitis.

If the stoma is friable and dusky after surgery, the surgeon may choose to be conservative and simply observe it for a while, hoping that reoperation is not necessary. One can insert a glass test tube through the stoma (Fig. 3-8),

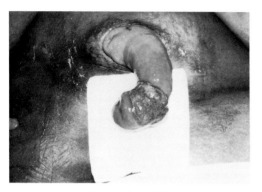

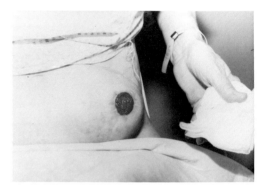

**Figure 3-9.** Prolapse of the distal end of a loop transverse colostomy. Note the trauma caused to the extended bowel by the pouch. (Reprinted with permission from J Enterostom Ther 11[1]: 37, 1984.[21])

**Figure 3-10.** Herniation around an end sigmoid colostomy.

with bowel function, the treatment consists of surgical revision. The surgeon may find that making a circumferential incision around the stoma, freeing the bowel to the fascial or peritoneal level, excising the stenotic terminal portion of the bowel, and advancing healthy intestine to make a new stoma is sufficient treatment. Otherwise, required treatment is a repeat laparotomy and possibly relocation of the stoma.

### Prolapse

Prolapse can affect end colostomies and both limbs of a loop colostomy (Fig. 3-9). What occurs is actually an intussusception of the proximal bowel through the colostomy stoma. Although the precise causes for prolapse remain unclear, predisposing factors include an excessively large aperture in the abdominal wall (this may result from making a stoma for a distended, edematous bowel), inadequate fixation of the bowel mesentery, or loss of fascial support at the stomal site from inadequate fixation or infection. An increase in intraabdominal pressure tends to exacerbate the problem. Once the process begins, it usually becomes progressively worse.

The surgeon can prevent this complication by not making the opening in the abdominal wall too large and by using sutures to attach the mesentery to the peritoneum and fascia. Mechanical bowel preparation, prophylactic antibiotics, and meticulous aseptic surgical technique with adequate hemostasis will, we hope, reduce the incidence of peristomal infection.

As long as the prolapse is mild, it may be tolerated as a nuisance. Most patients quickly learn to reduce the prolapsed segment by lying down and gently pushing the bowel back in place. A cold wash cloth over the stoma may help. A binder applied while the stoma is reduced may keep the bowel in place. We do not recommend a belted or hard-ringed colostomy appliance because the bowel can push out against the hard ring. The opening in the appliance should be large enough to accommodate the prolapsed bowel without constricting it or abrading the mucosa. The patient must be careful to protect the exposed bowel from trauma.

If the prolapse is severe, or if it becomes edematous and incarcerated, surgical revision is indicated. Prolapse of an end colostomy that has not progressed over a period of time may be corrected by simply circumferentially incising the stoma, dissecting the bowel from the surrounding tissue down to the fascia or peritoneum, amputating the excess length, and reestablishing the stoma. When the prolapse is progressive, however, the surgeon must reoperate and suture the mesentery and bowel wall to the peritoneum and fascia. If a loop colostomy is prolapsing, it may have to be converted to an end colostomy and mucous fistula. If the abdominal wall aperture is too large or if a concurrent parastomal hernia is present, the stoma should be relocated.

### Parastomal Hernia

Some degree of herniation is common, especially for an end colostomy (Fig. 3-10). This complication occurs when the stoma is placed in the abdominal incision or when the fascial incision is too large. Infection also leads to the development of a hernia. As intraabdominal pressure increases, the tendency towards herniation may be accentuated. As with prolapse, once begun, the hernia may enlarge progressively. It may contain colon, small intestine, or omentum. A large bulge makes an intact appliance fit almost impossible. Irrigation becomes difficult if a loop of colon is trapped between the fascia and the skin. The water may not go in or, once it does go in, it may not come out. Patients who use catheters to irrigate their colostomy should switch to a cone if they develop a hernia,[10] since catheters can perforate the bowel folded within the hernia. The best precaution is to have patients stop irrigating and manage their colostomy with a drainable pouch.

Preventive surgical techniques include making the opening in the abdominal wall as small as possible and keeping the stoma out of the incision. It is common surgical practice to bring the colostomy out through the middle of the rectus abdominis muscle for stability. Some surgeons suggest that bringing the colostomy out through the umbilicus will reduce herniation. We do not recommend this for patients with cancer because, at some future date, they may require additional surgery to manage either tumor recurrence or treatment complications.

Many hernias are asymptomatic and are tolerated as a nuisance. An incarcerated parastomal hernia, however, can result in intestinal obstruction or gangrene, therefore becoming a surgical emergency. Surgical repair consists of dissecting the colostomy from the surrounding tissue, excising the hernia sac, repairing the hernia defect, and relocating the stoma. Attempts at maintaining the same colostomy site are doomed to fail.

### Suture Separation

Sutures may separate if the suture line is under tension, the tissue is friable, or the blood supply is compromised. If separation occurs immediately after surgery, the sutures may be replaced. If the mucosal tissue is already attached to the fascia and subcutaneous tissue, however, the stoma may be allowed to granulate and heal by secondary intention. This usually results in a smaller stoma. Patients should be observed for stricture after the stoma has healed.

### Hemorrhage

Early postoperative hemorrhage is almost always the result of inadequate hemostasis. This complication can be obviated by simply maintaining meticulous hemostasis at the time of stomal construction. Later causes of stomal bleeding include skin or mucosal ulceration from colostomy excretions, trauma from the appliance, stomal varices in a patient with portal hypertension, or recurrent neoplasm at the stomal site. A patient with thrombocytopenia due to recent chemotherapy or radiotherapy may also develop stomal hemorrhage, although this occurs rarely.

For a patient with cancer, investigative studies should include a coagulation profile. If severe thrombocytopenia is present, platelet transfusions may be required. Local treatment should consist of ligating or cauterizing bleeding vessels.

### Separation of the Bowel Over a Bridge

The bridge or rod used to support the bowel in a loop colostomy can actually serve as a saw and sever the bowel if it is under too much tension over the bridge. If this occurs soon after surgery, the bowel may retract back into the abdominal wall; in this instance, surgical intervention is necessary.

### Peristomal Infection or Abscess

In our experience with cancer patients, even those who have received abdominal or pelvic radiotherapy, peristomal infection or abscess is surprisingly rare. Predisposing factors include nonsterile surgical technique, inadequate hemostasis, and placement of fixating sutures through the entire thickness of bowel wall. A peristomal abscess may be prevented by avoiding these errors in surgical technique. As for any abscess, treatment should consist of incision and drainage. Consequent stomal distortion may later necessitate reconstruction or relocation.

### Perforation

Perforation of the colostomy is a serious complication and requires surgical intervention. It may be manifested by an acute onset of pain next to the stoma accompanied by redness and swelling, and fever. Diffuse abdominal pain may also be present.

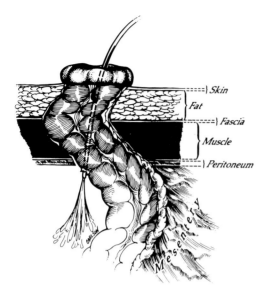

Skin
Fat
Fascia
Muscle
Peritoneum

**Figure 3-11.** Perforation of the bowel wall may occur during irrigation when the fascia and skin openings are not aligned.

The most common cause of bowel perforation in a patient with a colostomy is trauma from a catheter inserted for an irrigation or a barium enema. Some of the older irrigation sets employed hard tubing, easily capable of perforation. An irrigation catheter hardened from age or a routine enema catheter is also stiff enough to cause perforation. If the fascia opening and skin opening are not directly in line with one another there can be a scissoring effect, and as the tubing goes through the fascia at an angle it can tear the bowel (Fig. 3-11). Or, as the patient ages, the bowel may settle into a slight hernia around the stoma, making entry into the colostomy difficult.

To prevent perforation, a very soft, flexible catheter or a cone should be used for irrigations and barium enemas. If the physician or nurse has any reason to suspect increased risk of perforation in a patient, i.e., the patient is elderly, debilitated, has developed visual or dexterity problems, or is complaining about difficulty with irrigation, the procedure should be stopped and the patient should be taught to manage his colostomy with a drainable pouch.

Perforation can result in significant mortality. Frequently the patient is elderly, may already have peritonitis from fecal spillage, and waits a day or two before seeking medical attention. Treatment of the perforation requires parastomal drainage and may also require a diversion proximal to the perforation.

### Recurrent Neoplasm

Although a relatively rare complication, recurrent or progressive cancer may cause a tumor mass to develop at or near the stoma site. If the tumor is small and asymptomatic and the patient's remaining life is predicted to be brief, no therapy may be indicated. If, on the other hand, all treatment options have not been exhausted and the patient's disease may still be cured or palliated, then surgical resection and stoma relocation may be indicated. Depending upon the specific clinical circumstances, chemotherapy or radiotherapy may be administered to reduce the tumor. If the tumor nodules are in the skin, the patient may need to use a skin barrier to minimize friction or trauma to the nodule. Patients who use a presized pouch can cut extra room in the opening to prevent ulceration at the stoma site.

### Skin Irritation

Skin irritation must be recognized and promptly treated. The most frequent causes of skin problems are, first, improper location of the stoma, resulting in an ill-fitting appliance and fecal leakage; second, infection; and third, allergies. Appropriate treatment for skin problems is discussed in Chapter 10.

## Care of the Colostomy

There is no one way to take care of a colostomy. Many important variables determine the method of care: the anatomic location of the opening in the bowel; the surgical construction (loop, end, decompression); the location of the stoma; and personal variables of the patient, i.e., age, dexterity, prior bowel habits, reason for colostomy, activity level, overall health, and need for further treatment.

### Immediate Postoperative Stoma Care

Immediately after surgery, in either the operating room or the recovery room, the colostomy stoma is fitted with a skin barrier and a clear, drainable, odor-proof pouch. Although fecal output has usually not begun at this time (unless the bowel has been obstructed or the patient has not undergone mechanical bowel

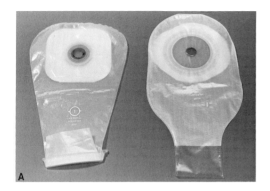

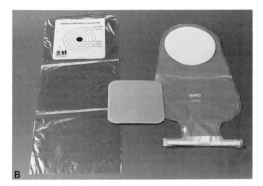

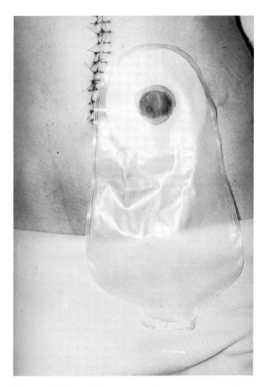

**Figure 3-12.** Colostomy pouches. **A,** one-piece precut drainable pouches that incorporate skin barriers in the adhesive (Hollister and Conva Tec). **B,** pouches that may be custom cut (United, Bard) and added to a skin barrier (Conva Tec).

**Figure 3-13.** With an end colostomy with a flush stoma, the wafer skin barrier is custom cut to fit closely around the stoma and away from the sutures, and a clean, drainable, odor-resistant pouch is applied over the skin barrier. (Reprinted with permission from Am J Nurs 85, [11]:1247, 1985.[20])

preparation), there may be serous or bloody drainage. The barrier and pouch protect the skin from irritation and keep the incisional dressings dry. Pouches used for colostomy care are almost exclusively disposable. Various one- and two-piece systems are available (Fig. 3-12). Some are precut and incorporate a skin barrier in the adhesive, and some may be custom cut and require a separate skin barrier. The main concern is to select an odor-proof pouch that provides a seal at the base of the stoma and does not allow fecal contents to remain on the skin or to undermine the adhesive of the pouch.

To prepare the skin around a new stoma, the nurse washes it gently with warm water and pats it dry, being careful not to put tension on the new sutures or to cause bleeding. If the patient has an end colostomy, round and flush, appliance selections include either a presized

pouch with skin barrier incorporated, a wafer skin barrier with a custom-cut pouch (Fig. 3-13), or a two-piece custom-cut system (Fig. 3-14). If the patient has a loop colostomy with a plastic rod or bridge under the bowel for support, a large two-piece custom-cut colostomy set or a large skin-barrier wafer and colostomy pouch are needed (Fig. 3-15). A small amount of skin-barrier paste can be applied over the rim of the bridge for a smoother surface and squeezed under and around the bridge as a filler to help make a seal. The opening in the skin barrier should be cut to the size of the stoma, covering the bridge. It is not a safe practice to incorporate the rod inside the opening and the pouch because of the possibility of pulling the bridge and tearing the bowel when removing the pouch.

A loop colostomy with a skin bridge or

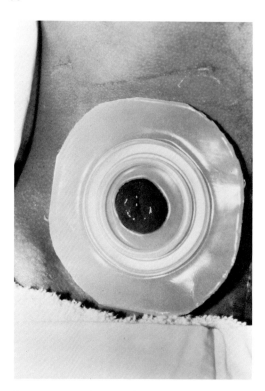

**Figure 3-14.** A two-piece custom-cut wafer that has a snap-on ring for the pouch. The wafer is cut to fit snugly around the stoma.

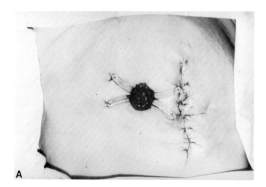

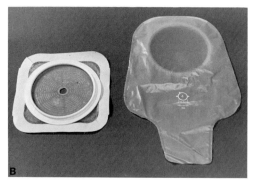

**Figure 3-15.** **A,** a loop descending colostomy over a plastic support bridge. (Reprinted with permission from Broadwell D, Appleby C, Bates M, Jackson B: Principles and techniques of pouching, in Broadwell D, Jackson B (Eds): Principles of Ostomy Care. St. Louis: The C. V. Mosby Co, 1982, p 578.[1]) **B,** a large two-piece loop ostomy set.

fascia bridge can be cared for like an end stoma, using a wafer skin barrier and pouch (one- or two-piece system) cut to the size of the stoma. If the edges of the stoma are irregular at the site of the skin bridge, a small amount of paste can serve as a filler. For a stoma in or near an incision, one can apply paste at the edge of the sutures (see Fig. 2-38). It does not interfere with the healing of the incision and provides a smooth surface for the skin barrier to adhere to. Paste and skin barrier on the incision are certainly preferable to stool leaking onto the incision! The wafer skin barrier and pouch cut to the size of the stoma can then be applied.

If the stoma is near another stoma, a wafer skin barrier can be cut small and the opening for the pouch cut off-center (Fig. 3-16) or, if needed, the two stomas can be placed within the same skin barrier and pouch. If the stoma is retracted, a small amount of paste at the edges of the stoma can fill in the creases; a flexible skin barrier and pouch can then fit securely. Presized pouches

with a hard ring usually do not work on a retracted stoma because the stool coming out of the stoma goes under the ring and breaks the seal of the adhesive. A severely retracted stoma may require a convex plate (see Chapter 2). For a stoma that has prolapsed, we prefer a soft skin barrier and flexible pouch, either a one-piece or two-piece custom-cut set. The opening must be large enough to keep it from rubbing against the bowel mucosa. A belt or hard rings should be avoided, because they provide resistance, causing the prolapse to increase.

As soon as the nurse has applied the pouch, he or she should record the first data about the stoma. Included are the color of the stoma; its size; whether it is nippled, flush, retracted, or prolapsed; the type of stoma—loop, end,

Turnbull, or mucous fistula; the condition of the skin; and the type of appliance used. These notes provide a basis for comparison so that other persons examining the stoma can detect changes or early signs of problems. Early postoperative problems to watch for are stoma necrosis, bleeding, suture separation, retraction, sloughing, prolapse, and skin irritation. Bleeding that can not be controlled by pressure, one or more sutures separating, or ischemia of the stoma may need immediate attention.

The stoma must be examined daily. In uncomplicated cases, we use a clear pouch and observe the stoma through it. Since the bowel may not resume functioning and the colostomy pass stool for several days, the skin barrier and pouch can remain intact during that time. However, when the stoma requires more careful observation because of ischemia or some other problem, we prefer a two-piece appliance so that we can remove the pouch and leave the skin barrier intact.

As the colostomy begins to function and the patient recovers from surgery, the nurse begins teaching colostomy care. Early lessons include how to empty the pouch, use a deodorant, and close the pouch again. In subsequent lessons the patient learns to remove the pouch, clean the stoma and skin, prepare a new pouch, and apply the pouch over the stoma. Patients who are candidates for regulation by colostomy irrigation may be taught the technique before discharge or on a return clinic visit, depending on their rate of recovery, speed of learning, and acceptance of responsibility for their care.

*Living with a Colostomy*

*Activity.* Persons with a colostomy should be encouraged to return to their normal activities after they have recovered from surgery. Unless there are unusual complications, patients are not limited in physical activities because of the colostomy. Patients can return to work and can swim, play golf or tennis, ride horseback, ski, and participate in other sports.

*Diet.* Foods that may influence colostomy function fall under four categories: gas-producing, including greens, beans, and onions; odor-causing—eggs, fish, cheeses, peas, greens, and cabbage; constipating—cheeses, bananas, tea,

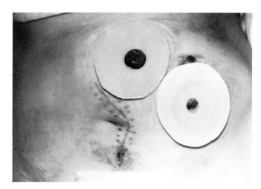

**Figure 3-16.** When the location of multiple stomas precludes using standard sized appliances, skin barriers and faceplates may need to be trimmed to fit.

and peanut butter; and purging—greens, fruit, prunes, beans, and cabbage.

For the first few days after surgery, patients with a colostomy take no nutrients by mouth. They begin oral intake with a clear liquid diet and progress to a full liquid, soft, and then a regular diet as their bowel function returns. Because the bowel is edematous from being handled and cut during surgery, we advise patients to avoid a lot of roughage and gas-forming foods for the first few days of eating. These foods add to distention and discomfort from gas. After patients have recovered from surgery, however, they should be encouraged to eat a normal diet.

Foods that have had a tendency to form gas, cause diarrhea, or cause constipation before surgery will have the same effect after surgery. Accordingly, patients usually want to select the times to eat these foods. For example, a patient may realize that beans cause gas for him, but beans are a favorite food and he does not want to omit them from his diet. He can choose to eat them, though, at a time when the uncontrollable passage of gas is not a nuisance for him. If another patient finds cheeses or peanut butter to be constipating, she may plan to counter their action by eating foods like bran, raisins, or prunes.

The best way for patients with a colostomy to manage their diet is to return to the style of eating and the lifetime habits that were theirs before the ostomy surgery.

*Odor.* Most patients are concerned about odor. However, pouches today are odor resistant, and the only time odor is detected is when stool or gas is escaping, either by leakage or because the pouch is open for emptying. A leaking pouch must be replaced. The practice of placing a pinhole in a pouch to let flatus out is self-defeating, because the pouch is then no longer odor resistant. Many pouches have a built-in charcoal-filtered vent to let flatus escape with minimal odor.

A number of methods are available to help patients reduce or control odor. For example, to counteract the strong odor that certain vitamin preparations and antibiotics cause in feces, patients can try ingesting buttermilk or yogurt. Other measures help to neutralize odor when the patient opens the pouch, such as spraying a small amount of ostomy deodorant in the room first, and spraying Peri-wash soap into a bedpan or container into which the pouch is emptied. This not only helps to absorb the odor, but also facilitates cleaning the container. After the pouch is emptied, spraying an ostomy soap and deodorant back into the pouch both neutralizes odor and keeps the feces from sticking to the pouch, making it easier to empty later. The same procedures help to control odor when the patient irrigates the colostomy: spraying an ostomy deodorant in the room first, spraying Peri-wash soap into the irrigation sleeve and spreading it around to coat the inside, and spraying Peri-wash and deodorant into the bedpan if it is used. The commode should be flushed or the bedpan emptied frequently during the procedure. Throughout the irrigation returns, the patient should rinse the sleeve frequently with a solution of warm water and ostomy soap or mouthwash.† While the sleeve is not being rinsed, its top should be folded over and clamped to keep odor from escaping in the patient's face.

Cleanliness is, of course, an essential requirement for odor control.

*Gas.* Voluntary control of the passage of flatus through a colostomy is not possible, since the stoma contains no sphincter. Patients soon learn which foods produce excessive flatus for

them and, although they do not have to completely eliminate these foods from their diet, they may select when they eat them.

Patients should be taught that flatus is increased by swallowing air, chewing gum, talking while eating, smoking, eating rapidly, drinking carbonated beverages, drinking through straws, and skipping meals.[18] Patients can usually anticipate the passage of flatus and can muffle the sound by placing their hand or arm over the stoma, moving away from others, or making a sound (clearing the throat, rearranging a chair). Levitt suggests that flatulence can be reduced by restricting the quantity of carbohydrates ingested and keeping the diet low in lactose, legumes, and wheat.[17] Some patients take antiflatulent tablets such as DiGel or Mylicon-80 orally to reduce flatus. One of the benefits of irrigation as a regulatory procedure is that it removes stool and flatus stored in the colon.

Patients with a colostomy tend to be extremely sensitive about gas and odor. The health care team should make every effort to teach the patient helpful techniques for control while at the same time not making a big issue out of these inconveniences. Reassuring statements, such as, "The passage of flatus is a natural function of every person," may help to minimize embarrassment. Team members should acknowledge patients' concerns, but help them respond to the uncontrolled passage of flatus matter-of-factly.

### Colostomy Irrigation

On the topic of colostomy irrigation, the literature is filled with a multitude of techniques, variations, "how tos," and "musts."[8,12,13,19,22,24,27] In this chapter we discuss irrigation for three basic purposes: bowel regulation, bowel preparation, and bowel stimulation. The purpose influences the method of irrigation used.

*Irrigation for bowel regulation.* When regulation is the goal, irrigation is performed solely for the patient's convenience. A healthy colostomy functions without irrigation. Forming a stoma does not interfere with bowel peristalsis after the patient has recovered from surgery. Therefore if regulatory irrigation becomes inconvenient for a patient, it should be stopped. The intent is to use the irrigation to stimulate the bowel to work at a specified time every day or every other day with little or no spillage of stool between irrigations. The patient can then wear a

---

† Mouthwash is a convenient deodorant if commercial deodorants are not available. It has a pleasant aroma and does not irritate the stoma.

small security pouch or stoma cap and not have to deal with much flatus or stool elimination throughout the day.

Not every person or every type of colostomy can function successfully with this method of care. People's bowel patterns are different, and can even vary from day to day. They are influenced by diet, medications, illness, emotions, and activities. Therefore when the physician or nurse is selecting a patient as a candidate for regulatory colostomy irrigation, he or she must evaluate a number of factors. First is the anatomic location of the colostomy. Ascending and transverse colostomies are usually unsuitable for regulation by irrigation because the stool is too liquid. Second, one must determine whether the bowel proximal to the ostomy has undergone any therapy. Bowel resection or radiotherapy may have increased the transit time of the bowel, which could cause stool spillage between irrigations. Third, the age of the patient is a factor. It is important that the patient be independent. A child should be old enough to perform the irrigation without assistance from his parents. An elderly adult, too, should be able to irrigate without help. If a person requires help with the irrigation, the resulting feelings of dependency outweigh the goals of convenience.

Prior bowel habits can provide a clue about how a patient will respond to irrigations. Some people have bowels that are easily stimulated, some have irritable bowels that evacuate two or three times a day, and some people have sluggish bowels that evacuate every two to three days. Life-long bowel habits usually do not change after colostomy surgery if most of the colon is intact. A person who has a history of several bowel movements a day will be difficult to restrict to one a day. Someone with a sluggish or constipated bowel can more easily achieve continence with irrigation.

The general health of the patient is a factor to consider. Does the patient have prospects of becoming more ill, for example with metastatic cancer? Is postoperative chemotherapy or radiotherapy being considered? Does the irrigation procedure leave the patient exhausted for the remainder of the day? Does the patient have diminished vision, arthritis, an intentional tremor, or an unhealed perineal wound that makes the irrigation procedure painful or burdensome? In these situations, regulatory irrigation may not be worthwhile.

Finally, personal preference may be the most important factor of all. Is the patient motivated to irrigate routinely, or would he prefer to manage his colostomy with a drainable pouch, emptying it as needed and changing it every three or four days?

If the physician or nurse has determined that a patient would like to try irrigating for regulation, appropriate lessons should be begun. A number of procedures are available for colostomy irrigation, one of which is cited in Appendix 3-1. The teacher must remember the goal of the irrigation—convenience—and keep the procedure as simple and as short as possible. The technique can and should be individualized; when results are not satisfactory, the patient should try some variations of technique. Patients should not become discouraged if irrigation does not regulate the colostomy right away. Several weeks may be needed for the bowel to recover from surgery and resume a regular pattern.

The first irrigation after surgery is given to most patients while they are in bed. Symptoms of nausea and weakness are not uncommon. The bowel may still be edematous and fairly inactive, so a small amount of water, 300–500 ml, is usually sufficient for the first irrigation. The water may or may not return, depending on the response of peristalsis in the bowel. If it does not, the nurse must be sure to record the amount instilled and to add it to the patient's amount of fluid intake.

As the patient improves, the lessons for colostomy irrigation should be transferred to the bathroom. The first time, this is difficult for most patients. If a patient has a perineal incision, pain medication administered before he gets out of bed may ease the trauma. The nurse should prepare the bathroom, have all of the equipment ready, and prepare a comfortable place for the patient to sit, for example a chair with a pillow, before getting the patient up. It is important to explain the procedure in advance and to perform it as smoothly and quickly as possible, so the patient is not out of bed too long for the first bathroom irrigation. The nurse should always stay with the patient, because he may become faint and nauseated and need assistance.

The timing of the colostomy irrigation is an individual matter based on the patient's previous bowel habits and daily living pattern at home and the time the colostomy is most active. Some patients may begin irrigating every day and then try to move to a schedule of every other day. Some patients irrigate in the morning before leaving for work, some wait until evening when there is less hurry and demand for bathroom facilities. Many patients find that irrigation is most effective after a meal. At first keeping to a fairly regular schedule is important, but after a time, slight variations may not matter.

*Irrigation for bowel preparation.* When irrigation is performed as preparation for a diagnostic procedure such as colonoscopy or barium enema, the goal is to empty the bowel contents from the colon; for a colonoscopy, the bowel walls must be really clean. The procedure differs, therefore, from a routine daily irrigation in that it requires more fluid and may have to be repeated several times. The process goes more rapidly if the patient has been limited to a restrictive diet the day before to reduce bowel residue (see Appendix 3-2).

The irrigation procedure itself is the same as that described in Appendix 3-1, except that it may need several repetitions. If a patient does not regularly irrigate his colostomy, the floor nurse or x-ray nurse should perform the irrigation. Patients who know how to irrigate their colostomy can do it themselves. They follow the prescribed dietary preparation during the day (Appendix 3-2). After dinner, they irrigate the colostomy with one quart of warm water, and repeat the irrigation at 6 A.M. on the day of the procedure. All patients should place a drainable colostomy pouch over their stoma after the morning irrigation and take an extra pouch with them to the x-ray department.

After a barium enema it is important that the barium be evacuated. Our usual procedure is to require the patient to drink at least four eight-ounce glasses of any liquid during the first eight hours after the enema. We ask the patient to irrigate the colostomy with one quart of water at bedtime and to take a mild laxative. If the stool is still chalky white the day after the examination, the patient should repeat the irrigation and again take a mild laxative (two ounces milk of magnesia). Patients who do not irrigate their colostomy should only take the laxative.

*Irrigation for constipation or impaction of stool or barium.* The purpose of this type of

irrigation is to remove impacted stool or barium from the colon. Impaction is a common problem for patients with cancer. Inactivity, pain medications, and some chemotherapy agents contribute to constipation. Barium, if not promptly removed after radiologic studies, can harden in the colon.

If the patient is mildly constipated, a regular irrigation of warm water may be sufficient to stimulate the bowel and cause a bowel movement. If the stool or barium has hardened, efforts must be directed toward breaking up the stool. Water alone just hits the stool and comes back out, causing cramping but few results. If this is the situation, an irrigation should be performed as a retention enema (Appendix 3-3), in small amounts, and repeated several times until the stool breaks up and is passing.

For a retention enema, 200–250 ml solution is instilled into the colostomy by a catheter or an irrigation set. It should go as high into the bowel as possible. A baby nipple or a dam helps to hold the solution in the bowel for a few minutes.

Several agents can be used as retention enema solutions. Each has advantages and disadvantages, and should be selected individually. The first, mineral oil, is a mild agent that does not cause cramping. However, it usually needs to be repeated several times, and does not stimulate peristalsis. Liquid colace helps to pull liquid into the colon but, like mineral oil, does not stimulate peristalsis, and is expensive to use. Liquid pericolace does help stimulate peristalsis, but it too is expensive to use. Fleet enema solution is stronger than mineral oil, colace, or pericolace. It stimulates peristalsis, but causes cramping. It is easy to administer; it comes in a prepackaged bulb that can be connected to a catheter with a baby nipple as a dam. A solution of milk and molasses pulls fluid into the bowel, stimulates peristalsis, and causes cramping. It is messy to administer, but frequently gets results. And finally, a soap suds solution, which is easy to prepare, has a detergent effect that breaks up stool and barium. However, it causes cramping and can irritate the lining of the bowel if used too frequently.

When selecting what type of solution to use for a retention enema, one should consider the specific problem, the acuteness of need, and the action of the various agents. If the patient has an obstruction or a recent bowel anastomosis, one should use a solution that does not stimulate peristalsis, which could perforate the colon or break down the anastomosis. If barium is visible on x-ray and the patient is not otherwise obstructed, a Fleet enema, milk and molasses, or a detergent may be necessary.

## ILEOSTOMY

### Historical Development

Scattered reports of ileostomies came from Europe in the late 1800s, but the first ileostomy in America was not performed until 1913.[3] The operation continued to be performed for the next 40 years, although with considerable morbidity and mortality.

One of the complications frequently encountered was ileostomy "dysfunction," a term designating partial obstruction at the stoma. In 1951, Warren and McKittrick[26] recognized the cause of this "dysfunction" and recommended longitudinal incisions through the seromuscular layers to relieve the problem. Crile and Turnbull[5] in this country and Brooke[2] in England also appreciated the nature of this problem in the early 1950s, and independently they devised procedures for alleviating it. Crile and Turnbull recommended the mucosal-grafted ileostomy: stripping the seromuscular layers of the stoma, everting the full-thickness bowel upon itself, and suturing it to the skin. This procedure has become the standard. Kock[15] introduced a continent ileostomy in 1965 that is becoming increasingly popular for selected patients.

### Indications

Probably the most common indication for ileostomy is inflammatory bowel disease—ulcerative colitis and Crohn's disease. However, in this chapter we restrict the discussion to indications related to cancer or a predisposition to developing cancer.

#### Familial Polyposis

Familial polyposis is an inherited form of intestinal polyposis in which benign polyps develop in the colon and rectum during the teenage years and then invariably undergo a carcinomatous change in the third or fourth decade. It is inherited as an autosomal dominant trait, and therefore appears in each successive generation.

It is more common in men than in women and is almost never diagnosed before puberty. The treatment of choice is total proctocolectomy and formation of an end ileostomy. For selected patients, some surgeons recommend colectomy and ileoproctostomy and close follow-up.

#### Gardner's Syndrome

Gardner first described the syndrome bearing his name in 1950.[11] This condition is also inherited as an autosomal dominant trait. It consists of multiple intestinal polyps with associated bone or connective-tissue tumors. In this condition also, colonic polyps have a strong tendency toward carcinomatous change. Treatment is similar to that for familial polyposis: either total proctocolectomy with an end ileostomy or colectomy and ileoproctostomy.

#### Carcinoma of the Colon

Although ileostomy is performed only rarely in patients with colon cancer, it is indicated in occasional circumstances. A patient who has cancer of the right side of the colon or the cecum associated with obstruction or perforation may require a primary resection with a temporary ileostomy and mucous fistula. In addition, a palliative ileostomy may be the best treatment for a patient with unresectable cancer of the right colon or cecum or with carcinomatosis arising from this area.

#### Carcinomatosis

The disease associated most frequently with carcinomatosis and intestinal obstruction is epithelial ovarian cancer. Approximately 25 percent of all patients with ovarian cancer develop an intestinal obstruction at some time in the course of their disease. This obstruction is usually related to progressive intraabdominal tumor growth and is a preterminal event. Many other types of cancer—endometrial, cervical, colonic, pancreatic, gastric, etc.—may, however, be associated occasionally with progressive carcinomatosis and intestinal obstruction. In these patients the initial treatment decision is whether or not a surgical procedure is indicated. Many factors influence this decision, including the surgeon's attitude toward and experience with cancer patients and the patient's general condition, anticipated survival time, and desire for surgery.

If surgery is performed in such patients, the

optimal procedure, of course, is resection of a localized obstructing lesion in the small bowel or colon and either primary reanastomosis or an intestinal bypass. Unfortunately, many of these patients have disseminated bulky tumor obstructing multiple areas of the colon and distal small intestine. In these patients, a palliative loop ileostomy or end ileostomy and mucous fistula may be created to relieve the obstruction and, the surgeon hopes, improve the quality of the patient's remaining life. Sometimes, however, even a palliative ileostomy is not possible. Then a tube gastrostomy may be performed to obviate a nasogastric tube and, perhaps, allow the patient to go home from the hospital.

### Radiation Injury to the Small Intestine

Radiotherapy, either whole-pelvis or abdominopelvic, can be the treatment of choice for a variety of cancers—cervical, endometrial, ovarian, and rectal. This treatment injures the small intestines of 5 to 10 percent of these patients, to an extent determined by field size, dosage, history of previous surgery, etc. The site most often injured is the terminal ileum.

When a small-intestinal injury is diagnosed, the treatment of choice is either intestinal resection with primary reanastomosis or intestinal bypass. If, however, diagnosis is delayed for whatever reason, intestinal obstruction may progress and lead to bowel necrosis and perforation. In such a situation, if gross peritoneal contamination is present, the treatment of choice should be resection of the necrotic segment of bowel and temporary construction of an end ileostomy and mucous fistula. At a later date, the ileostomy may be taken down and the reanastomosis accomplished under less contaminated conditions.

### Enterocutaneous Fistula

Very rarely, for selected patients with enterocutaneous fistulas and associated unresectable intraabdominal tumor, severe radiation fibrosis, or both, we have performed a diverting ileostomy proximal to the fistula site. Our hope is that the procedure will allow the fistula to heal spontaneously with the aid of intravenous hyperalimentation and skin protection while we treat the primary cancer, e.g., with chemotherapy. If the fistula closes spontaneously, then the ileostomy can be closed at a later date. This

unconventional treatment strategy has occasionally been successful in our patients.

## Preoperative Preparation

If time allows (i.e., an emergency indication for surgery does not exist), the patient is usually admitted to the hospital a few days prior to surgery. If the patient is malnourished, then a longer preoperative hospitalization may be indicated for intravenous hyperalimentation.

Prior to surgery the patient undergoes a mechanical and antibiotic bowel preparation. In our practice, most patients have already been evaluated clinically and by the indicated laboratory and radiologic studies. The stoma site is selected by the surgeon and the nurse (see Chapter 1).

We also use the preoperative period to provide patient and family education. The nursing staff becomes acquainted with the patient and begins to establish a relationship based on mutual honesty, trust, and respect. Problem areas are identified and support and information are provided. In addition, the nursing and social work staffs begin to formulate plans for postoperative and discharge care.

The social worker interviews patients and their families and identifies potential problem areas. The dietician evaluates the patient's nutritional status and makes recommendations for both preoperative nutrition and postoperative dietary management. The nurse and physician provide information about the type of stoma, its location, and the type of appliance to be worn. The patient and the health care team talk about the effect the stoma may have on the patient's daily life (i.e., clothing, bathing, exercise, swimming, personal relationships, and sex).

## Ileostomy Construction

The three major types of ileostomy currently used are end ileostomy, loop ileostomy, and continent or Kock ileostomy (Fig. 3-17). We do not discuss the latter in this chapter because this type of ileostomy is rarely indicated in patients who have cancer.

### The End Ileostomy

Early ileostomies frequently had the problem of "dysfunction" caused by partial obstruction at the stoma site itself. Improvements in

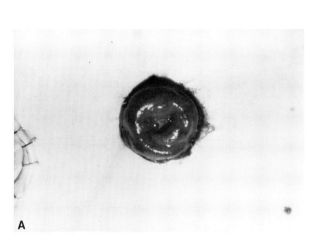

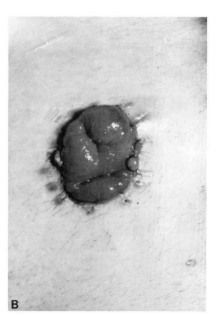

**Figure 3-17.** **A**, an end ileostomy constructed with a bud stoma. **B**, a loop ileostomy stoma. The proximal limb protrudes farther than the distal limb to throw the effluent out into the pouch, minimizing contact of the effluent with the skin.

technique made in the 1950s by Warren and McKittrick,[26] Crile and Turnbull,[5] and Brooke[2] have almost completely alleviated this problem. The Brooke technique, or modifications thereof, seems to be the procedure employed most often.

The surgeon selects an incision that is not too close to the stoma site and chooses the segment of intestine to be used to construct the ileostomy. Whether or not a resection (colectomy or small-bowel resection) is performed, the mesentery of the ileum should be divided in a manner that ensures an adequate blood supply to the terminal ileum while allowing sufficient mobility. Special problems encountered in mobilizing the ileal segment include a fixed, retracted mesentery caused by either tumor or radiation fibrosis. Adequate mobilization may also be a problem in an obese patient.

Next, the abdominal wall aperture is prepared (Fig. 3-18). The assistant grasps the fascia with a Kocher clamp and the skin with an Allis clamp and pulls these tissues medially to align the layers of the abdominal wall, thereby ensuring a vertical incision through it and avoiding a scissoring effect. Concurrently, the surgeon grasps the previously marked stoma site with a Kocher clamp and makes a circumferential incision 2 to 3 cm in diameter. The underlying subcutaneous tissue and fascia are then incised vertically, exposing the rectus abdominis muscle. After obtaining hemostasis, the surgeon bluntly separates the muscle with a clamp and makes an opening in the peritoneum wide enough to admit two fingers. A slightly larger stomal opening may be necessary in an obese patient.

The surgeon then grasps the end of ileum with a Babcock clamp and gently draws it through the abdominal wall aperture (Fig. 3-19A), being careful not to twist the mesentery. It is important to have at least 6 cm of ileum above the skin surface whenever possible. Next, the mesentery is sutured to the parietal peritoneum to prevent volvulus or internal hernia. Some surgeons prefer also to secure the bowel wall to the rectus fascia by placing a few interrupted sutures of 3-0 silk or Dexon between the fascia and the serosa of the ileum, taking care not to penetrate the full bowel wall thickness or damage the mesentery (Fig. 3-19B).

The main abdominal incision is then closed, and the surgeon completes the construction of

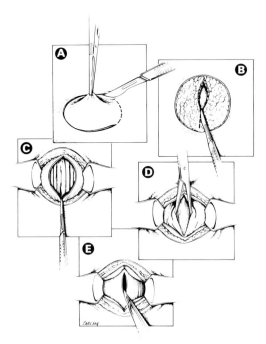

**Figure 3-18.** Construction of the abdominal wall aperture for an end ileostomy. **A**, the physician grasps the stoma site with a Kocher clamp and makes a circumferential incision. **B**, the incision in the subcutaneous tissue. **C**, the incision in the fascia. **D**, the rectus muscle is exposed. **E**, an opening is made in the peritoneum.

the stoma. First the mesentery of the ileum that protrudes above the skin level is resected. The clamp across the end of the bowel is then removed and the bleeding vessels ligated with 3-0 plain catgut. The surgeon everts the stoma, using clamps or sutures, and sutures the full thickness of bowel wall to the surrounding skin with interrupted 3-0 plain catgut. In obese patients, the thickness of the abdominal wall and the increased amount of mesenteric adipose tissue increase the likelihood of stomal complications. As noted above, the abdominal wall aperture may need to be made larger than normal to accommodate the excess tissue. In such a patient one should consider a modification of the end ileostomy—the J-loop ileostomy. In this procedure the stomal end is closed in two layers and a segment of intestine just proximal to the end is pulled through the aperture, incised, and sutured to the surrounding skin as described above (Fig. 3-20).

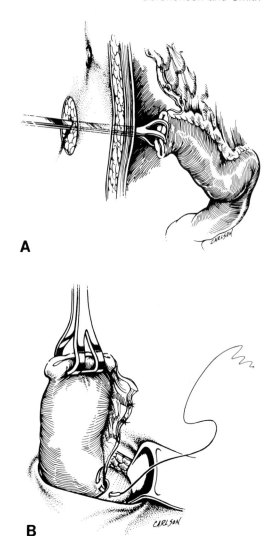

**Figure 3-19.** Technique for an end ileostomy. **A**, the end of the ileum is delivered through the abdominal wall aperture with a Babcock clamp. **B**, the seromuscular layers of the ileal wall are affixed to the fascia with interrupted sutures. Then, the protruding mesentery of the ileum is resected, and the ileal wall is everted and approximated to the skin with interrupted sutures of 3-0 plain catgut.

### The Loop Ileostomy

The standard permanent ileostomy is the end ileostomy. Under certain conditions, however, construction of an end ileostomy may not be possible, or even desirable. Such clinical situations might include, for example, the ileostomy performed to relieve intestinal obstruction in the debilitated patient with ovarian cancer and a short survival expectation.

To perform a loop ileostomy, the surgeon employs the same type of incision and method of constructing the abdominal wall aperture as is used for an end ileostomy. The only difference is that the aperture may need to be somewhat larger to accommodate the loop. The surgical steps for constructing a loop ileostomy are similar to those already described for a loop colostomy (Figs. 3-2 through 3-4). In beginning the loop ileostomy, the surgeon places a clamp just beneath the selected segment of intestine in an avascular space and passes an umbilical tape or Penrose drain through this space, encircling the bowel, to provide traction. He then pulls the loop gently through the abdominal wall aperture. A bridge is usually placed under the bowel to support the stoma, although an alternative is to develop a skin bridge. Next, the surgeon makes a transverse incision in the intestinal serosa and carries it through to the lumen. The mucosa is sutured to the skin with interrupted 3-0 plain catgut and, seven to ten days postoperatively, the bridge is removed.

## Complications

### Stomal Complications

Ileostomy complications can be divided into two types—stomal and metabolic. As any experienced surgeon is well aware, stomal complications are usually the result of either poor selection of a stomal site or errors in surgical technique. It is far preferable to spend a little longer time in constructing a healthy stoma, even if it means completely revising a stoma after a first inadequate attempt, than it is for both the patient and surgeon to suffer the consequences of a stomal complication, e.g., another surgical procedure.

Obviously, certain patients present a greater challenge to the surgeon. Obesity or the presence of multiple skin folds or previous abdominal incisions can surely make the construction of a proper stoma much more difficult. Moreover, patients with cancer often possess additional characteristics that are associated with a higher risk of stomal problems, such as intraperitoneal tumor, a history of prior radio-

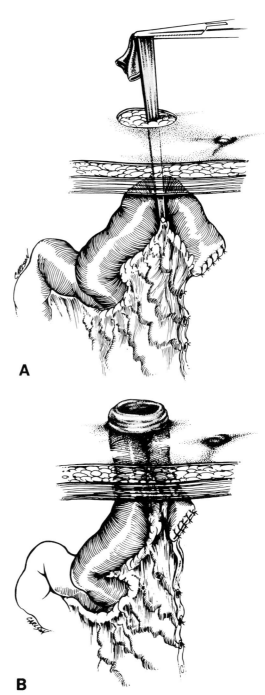

**A**

**B**

**Figure 3-20.** J-loop ileostomy. **A,** the segment of ileum proximal to the closed end of the bowel is delivered through the stomal aperture. **B,** an incision is made in the ileum, and the bowel wall is approximated to the skin edges with interrupted sutures of 3-0 plain catgut.

therapy or chemotherapy, or an immunosuppressed status. The oncologic surgeon must, therefore, take even greater care in the preoperative preparation and operative construction of the stoma.

Each stomal complication discussed for colostomies in this chapter is applicable to an ileostomy stoma. Three additional complications that may accompany an ileostomy stoma are fistula formation, ileostomy dysfunction, and obstruction.

*Fistula formation.* Although peristomal abscess and fistula formation occur relatively often in patients with inflammatory bowel disease, a peristomal fistula is exceedingly rare in a patient with cancer and an ileostomy. If it does occur, it is usually a result of placing the sutures used to fix the bowel wall to the fascia through the entire thickness of the bowel into the lumen. During stomal construction, the surgeon must be careful to place these sutures through only the seromuscular coat of the intestine. If a peristomal fistula occurs, maintaining a good seal of the appliance may be difficult, and skin excoriation may be the result. Although these fistulas occasionally heal spontaneously, they usually require surgical intervention, including reconstruction and relocation of the ileostomy stoma.

*Ileostomy dysfunction.* Ileostomy dysfunction is an occurrence of a large output of ileal effluent shortly after surgery. This complication was very common until the 1950s, when Crile and Turnbull of the Cleveland Clinic realized that the dysfunction was actually due to a partial obstruction at the stomal level.[5] The method used to construct the ileostomy stoma at that time left the serosa exposed and unprotected, serositis occurred, and the ileum became inflamed and edematous, causing a partial obstruction. Crile and Turnbull excised the seromuscular layer and everted the bowel on itself to protect the serosal surface. This procedure eliminated the problem of dysfunction and created a stoma that did not have alternating peristalsis. Its disadvantage, however, was that it was surgically difficult to construct.

Brooke[2] of England devised another technique to eliminate dysfunction: he everted the full thickness of the bowel on itself and sutured it to the abdominal skin, thus preventing the serositis and subsequent edema.

*Obstruction.* Several situations can cause intestinal obstruction in a patient with an ileostomy. It is of utmost importance to distinguish between those causes that require surgery and those that do not.

Almost all patients who have an ileostomy occasionally develop an obstruction caused by a particle or bolus of food. The result is a reduced output from the ileostomy and, frequently, cramps and nausea. This kind of obstruction may occur from kernels of popcorn, vegetable or fruit fiber, Chinese foods, nuts, corn, tough meat, or other poorly digestible foods; it appears most often in patients with a stricture or stenosis at the skin level. If the stoma begins to swell, the patient should remove the faceplate to prevent trauma to the stoma. Sometimes patients can dislodge their own food bolus by getting into the knee-chest position and massaging the abdomen. A warm bath may help, or the bolus may be relieved by digital probing.

If these efforts do not dislodge the obstruction, a physician or trained nurse can lavage the ileostomy stoma. To lavage the stoma, one must insert a 22-F or 24-F catheter, gently irrigate with 100 to 200 ml saline, and then remove the catheter. By observing the effluent, one can see if the bolus passes. If not, the lavage should be repeated until the blockage is removed. The patient may require hospitalization and intravenous fluid replacement after a food blockage. If no food particles appear in the lavage returns, the obstruction may have another cause, such as recurrent disease or adhesions. Lavage is not useful in these situations.

Other more serious causes of obstruction, which generally require surgical intervention, include internal herniation around the stoma, a volvulus, or intussusception. Cancer patients are at a high risk of developing a small bowel obstruction. Progressive tumor may lead to recurrent obstruction, especially in patients who have ovarian cancer or other cancers that metastasize to the abdomen. Patients who have received radiotherapy to the abdomen or pelvis are also prone to develop a small bowel obstruction. These are patients with cervical cancer, ovarian cancer, endometrial cancer, bladder cancer, or colon cancer. Of course, any patient who has had one or more operations may develop adhesions that can lead to obstruction.

*Metabolic Complications*

*Ileostomy diarrhea.* In the early postoperative period, a new ileostomy may produce as much as one to two liters of effluent per day. The amount of effluent produced during this period varies, depending on the type of ileostomy, previous ileal resection, or previous radiotherapy. When the ileostomy becomes established, this effluent usually decreases to a daily volume of less than one liter and contains approximately 120 mEq/l sodium and 500 ml water. In compensation, urine volume and urinary sodium excretion decrease.

Ileostomy diarrhea is defined as a daily effluent greater than 1000 ml. As daily volume increases, loss of water and sodium becomes excessive. In extreme cases, potassium and magnesium may also become depleted and metabolic acidosis may occur.

The major causes of ileostomy diarrhea may be divided into two categories, acute and chronic. Acute causes include infection, exposure to high temperatures, diuretic therapy, and partial obstruction. Thanks to modern surgical techniques, partial obstruction at the stomal site is rare unless it is due to a food bolus, discussed above. In treating acute ileostomy diarrhea, the physician should determine and alleviate the basic cause. Bacterial enteritis may require antibiotic therapy; viral gastroenteritis needs only symptomatic treatment. Some drugs used to treat cancer, such as cisplatin and metoclopramide, may cause temporary ileostomy diarrhea.

Supportive measures include oral administration of water and sodium when the diarrhea is mild. One must remember, however, that excessive salt intake (greater than 15 g per day) of itself leads to ileostomy diarrhea. Commercially available solutions such as Gatorade may be consumed to increase salt intake. Severe cases may require hospitalization and intravenous administration of fluid and electrolytes. If metabolic acidosis is present, administration of sodium bicarbonate may be indicated.

The chronic causes of ileostomy diarrhea— a history of ileal resection or radiotherapy— present a greater challenge to the clinician. These conditions tend to be constant and require meticulous care. In addition to the supportive measures described above, patients usually require chronic treatment with antidiarrheal agents such as tincture of opium, codeine, Lomotil, or loperamide. These drugs should be prescribed first at a normal dosage and then increased until the desired effect (decreased effluent) is achieved. Many patients require extremely high doses to control diarrhea.

When diarrhea is severe, the normal ileostomy pouch may be too small to contain the large volume of effluent; patients may need to use a bedside drainage bag. Vitamin B-12 absorption may also be impaired in these patients. If so, they may need monthly vitamin B-12 injections. For refractory cases, the surgeon should consider an antiperistaltic ileal segment. Several reports have documented acceptable results with this procedure.

*Urolithiasis.* Renal calculi occur in 6% to 10 percent of patients with an ileostomy, far more than in the normal population. The acid urine excreted by these patients may promote precipitation of uric acid crystals. Preventive measures consist of increased fluid intake to increase urine volume, antidiarrheal agents, if necessary, to decrease excessive ileostomy output, and oral sodium bicarbonate to alkalinize the urine.

*Cholelithiasis.* Most studies indicate that the incidence of cholelithiasis is very high in patients with ileostomies. Moreover, the incidence is directly proportional to the length of time the patient has had the ileostomy. Ileal resection has an adverse effect on the enterohepatic circulation with a consequent loss of bile acids in the stool. Although cholic acid preparations may be administered orally to prevent this complication, they may irritate the colon and produce severe diarrhea. When a patient with an ileostomy develops cholelithiasis, cholecystectomy may be indicated.

## Ileostomy Management

*Stomal Care*

The surgical construction of an ileostomy is not a common treatment for patients with a malignancy. There are probably as many colostomies that, because of radiotherapy or bowel resection, function as ileostomies as there are anatomically true ileostomies. If the colostomy stoma functions as an ileostomy, i.e., discharges liquid effluent, it must be managed in the same manner as an ileostomy.

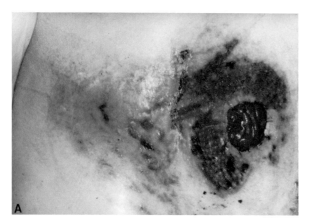

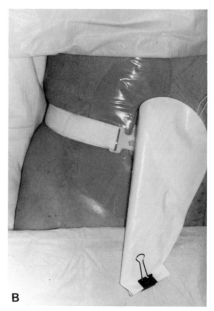

**Figure 3-21.** **A,** irritant contact dermatitis was caused by leakage of ileal effluent from an ileostomy. This severe dermatitis occurred after the appliance had leaked during the night and was not changed until morning. Note the diffuse erythema, edema, ulcerations, and oozing. **B,** a convex face plate and reusable ileostomy appliance are applied with an extended wafer or skin barrier over the area of dermatitis.

Because an ileostomy does not have the anatomic variables of a colostomy, its method of management is fairly constant. Appliance selection is influenced by the location and type of stoma. The principles are the same as those of the urinary stoma, discussed in Chapter 2. Both disposable and reusable appliances are suitable for an ileostomy as long as the pouch selected is odor-resistant and drainable. The major difference in the appliance management of an ileostomy stoma is the constant need for a skin barrier. The effluent from the ileum is caustic to the skin and can quickly cause erosion and maceration. The appliance must be carefully fitted to prevent effluent from undermining the adhesive. If any leakage does occur, the appliance must be completely removed and the skin cleaned immediately. Patching the edge of a leaking ileostomy pouch with tape for a few hours can result in serious skin problems (Fig. 3-21).

In the immediate postoperative period, the patient may be fitted with a clear disposable pouch with a skin barrier and/or paste next to

the stoma (Fig. 3-22). The pouch should be turned to the side to facilitate emptying by the staff. Depending on the length of time before bowel function returns, it may be several days before ileal effluent drains from the stoma. The first drainage is usually dark green and liquid. The effluent may eventually thicken to a pasty consistency as the patient resumes a normal diet. After patients become ambulatory and begin to assume some of the responsibility for caring for their ileostomy, the appliance should be turned downward. At this time the nurse should fit patients with the type of appliance they will wear at home and should begin teaching self-care (Chapters 2 and 5).

### Living with an Ileostomy

*Activity.* After they have recovered from surgery, patients need not limit their activity because of the ileostomy. Active sports, swimming, bathing, and travel are permissible. Before swimming or engaging in sports, the patient should check the security of the pouch. Waterproof tapes are available to provide added security for swimming. When traveling, patients should pack adequate supplies for the trip. From experience, we suggest that not all supplies be in checked luggage; patients should carry some with them in case luggage is lost or delayed.

*Diet.* After surgery, if the remaining small bowel is normal and capable of the same digestion and absorption as before, the patient need not strictly adhere to a bland diet. The only digestive change is the absence of water and electrolyte resorption in the colon, and eventually the small intestine takes over some of this function. Dietary caution is useful mainly for symptomatic relief of gas, odor, or diarrhea, and any restrictions are voluntary. Food eaten hurriedly and not chewed well may pass through as a mass and cause a blockage, but any food that is chewed thoroughly is permissible. At first, ileostomy patients are salt and water wasters; therefore an increase in salt and water in the diet is recommended to offset these losses. If a situation arises that increases sodium loss, such as excessive sweating or diarrhea, salt depletion is a possibility.

*Odor.* The problem of odor is contained by using odor-resistant pouches. There should be no odor unless the pouch is opened for emptying or has a hole or a leak. Commercial ostomy deodorants are available to use when emptying the pouch. The suggestions for colostomy care in this chapter are applicable to ileostomy care as well.

*Gas.* Although patients who have an ileostomy have no more gas after surgery than they did before, the effects of the flatus are more noticeable and socially embarrassing because of lack of control. Patients can take preventive measures to reduce the amount of air swallowed, which helps reduce gas. Since rapid eating, talking while eating, and gum chewing increase the amount of swallowed air, these should be avoided. Carbonated beverages produce gas, and anxiety contributes to gas formation. Patients usually have more gas postoperatively, while still in the hospital, than they do later. After the edema from surgery subsides and patients go home and resume their normal routine and eating habits, the amount of gas usually decreases.

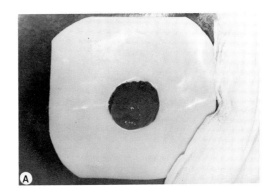

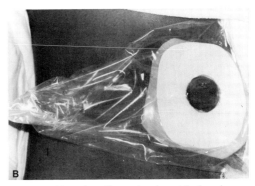

**Figure 3-22.** **A**, a Stomahesive skin-barrier wafer is cut to fit snugly next to the ileostomy stoma. **B**, a clear, drainable, odor-resistant pouch is applied postoperatively to an ileostomy stoma.

## CONCLUSION

Bowel diversions are becoming more common for patients with malignancies as surgical technique and ostomy management advance. A colostomy or ileostomy should no longer be considered a handicap or a "treatment worse than the disease." Whether the goal of the bowel diversion is full recovery or palliation, the goals for treating patients include their physical and emotional comfort, ability to manage their own ostomy, and return to their former life-style.

## APPENDIX 3-1

### Procedure for Colostomy Irrigation (Fig. 3-23)

1. Select an irrigation set with a cone or soft catheter and a dam.
2. Fill the irrigation container with 1000–1200 ml warm water.

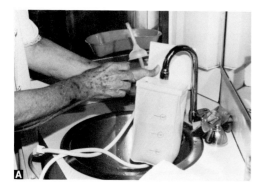
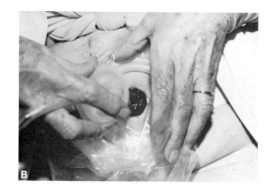
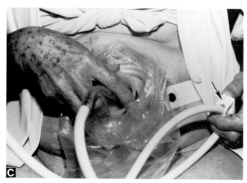
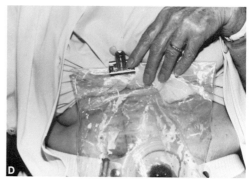

**Figure 3-23.** Steps in colostomy irrigation. **A,** an irrigation set with a soft catheter and dam, which the patient is filling with warm tap water. She lubricates the catheter tip with a water-soluble jelly and, **B,** she inserts the catheter tip gently into the stoma through the top of the irrigation sleeve. **C,** she controls the water flow with the clamp (arrow) while she supports the dam in the stoma. **D,** before allowing the effluent to return, she clamps the top of the irrigation sleeve.

3. Run the water through the tubing to expel the air.

4. Remove the used pouch or stoma cap.

5. Fasten the irrigation sleeve around the waist with the bottom of the sleeve in the commode.

6. Spray an ostomy deodorant in the room and some ostomy soap into the irrigation sleeve. This absorbs some of the odor and facilitates cleaning the sleeve.

7. Lubricate the tip of the cone or catheter with a water-soluble jelly.

8. Gently insert the cone or soft catheter two to three inches into the stoma, letting the water run slowly to open the bowel. Use a dam to keep the water from spilling back around the catheter. If it is inserted too far, there is a danger of perforating the colon. Also the water goes high into the bowel and

takes longer to return, adding time but no purpose to the irrigation.

9. Slowly let the water run in (approximately five minutes). If cramping occurs, slow or stop the water for a few seconds. It is not necessary to use all of the water; 500 ml is enough for a good irrigation for some persons.

10. After the water is instilled, remove the cone or catheter and close the top of the irrigation sleeve.

11. If the return flow is slow, massage the abdomen, clamp the bottom of the sleeve, and move around, drink a hot liquid, or gently pour warm water over the stoma.

12. After the irrigation, wash and dry the stoma and skin and apply a clean pouch or stoma cap.

13. Wash equipment with soap and water.

## APPENDIX 3-2

### Dietary Preparation for Barium Enema

*The day before the test:*
*12 p.m. (noon), Lunch*
 1 cup clear broth with crackers
 2 plain white-meat chicken or turkey sandwiches (no butter, lettuce, or other additive)
 $\frac{1}{2}$ glass (4 oz) clear apple or grape juice
 1 serving ($\frac{1}{2}$ cup) plain gelatin dessert (no cream, fruit, or other additive)
 1 glass (8 oz) skim milk

*1 p.m.*
 1 glass (8 oz) or more water

*3 p.m.*
 1 glass (8 oz) or more water

*5 p.m., Dinner*
 1 cup clear broth
 1 glass (8 oz) clear apple or grape juice
 1 serving ($\frac{1}{2}$ cup) plain gelatin dessert (no cream, fruit, or other additive)

*6 p.m.*
 1 glass (8 oz) or more water

*7 p.m.*
 $\frac{1}{2}$ bottle magnesium citrate (cold)

*Take nothing by mouth after midnight.*

## APPENDIX 3-3

### Procedure for Retention Enema

1. Apply an irrigation sleeve or a wide-mouth open-ended drainable pouch to the stoma.
2. Put the enema solution in an irrigation set or a disposable Fleet enema bottle.
3. Use an irrigation catheter with a dam or a soft catheter with a baby nipple for a dam.
4. Lubricate the catheter.
5. Insert the catheter through the top of the sleeve or through the bottom of the open-ended pouch.
6. Gently insert the catheter into the stoma as far as it will go.
7. Position the dam or nipple into the stoma to prevent back-flow.
8. Slowly run the solution into the bowel.
9. Hold the catheter and dam in place several minutes to keep the solution in the bowel.
10. Remove the catheter.
11. Close the bottom of the pouch or the sleeve top.

Fluid return is usually not immediate. This procedure may have to be repeated twice a day over several days if the stool or barium is severely impacted.

## REFERENCES

1. Broadwell D, Appleby C, Bates M, Jackson B: Principles and techniques of pouching, in Broadwell D, Jackson B (Eds): Principles of Ostomy Care. St. Louis, C. V. Mosby, 1982, pp 565–643
2. Brooke BN: The management of ileostomy including its complications. Lancet 2:102–104, 1952
3. Brown JY: The value of complete physiological rest of the large bowel in the treatment of certain ulcerative and obstructive lesions of this organ; with description of operative technique and report of cases. Surg Gynecol Obstet 16:610–613, 1913
4. Cheselden W: Anatomy of the Human Body. London, Livingston, 1784
5. Crile G Jr, Turnbull RB Jr: Mechanism and prevention of ileostomy dysfunction. Ann Surg 140:459–466, 1954
6. Devlin HB: The structure and function of a colostomy, in Walker FC (Ed): Modern Stoma Care. London, Churchill Livingstone, 1976, pp 41–67
7. Dinnick T: The origins and evolution of colostomy. Br J Surg 22:142–143, 1934
8. Doran J, Hardcastle JD: A controlled trial of colostomy management by natural evacuation, irrigation, and foam enema. Br J Surg 68:731–733, 1981
9. Drobni S, Icnze F: Historical Sketch: Surgery of Rectal Cancer. Budapest, Akademiai Kiado, 1969, pp 11–18
10. Gambrell E: The newer cones: Simple solution for water retention problems. Ostomy Quarterly 9(4):47, 1972
11. Gardner EJ, Richards RC: Multiple cutaneous and subcutaneous lesions occurring simulta-

neously with hereditary polyposis osteomatosis. Am J Hum Genet 5:139–147, 1953

12. Goode PS: Colostomy irrigation, in Broadwell D, Jackson B (Eds): Principles of Ostomy Care. St. Louis, C. V. Mosby, 1981, pp 369–380

13. Grier WRN, Postel AH, Syarse A: An evaluation of colonic stoma management without irrigation. Surg Gynecol Obstet 118:1234–1242, 1964

14. Kelsey CB: Surgery of the Rectum and Pelvis. New York, Richard Kettles and Company, 1897, p 315

15. Kock NG: Intraabdominal "reservoir" in patients with permanent ileostomy. Arch Surg 99:223–231, 1969

16. Kodner I: Colostomy and ileostomy. Clin Symp 30(5):2–36, 1978

17. Levitt M: Intestinal gas production: Recent advances in flatology. N Engl J Med 302:1474–1475, 1981

18. Martin PJ, Spratt JS: Stomas and their care, in Spratt JS (Ed): Neoplasms of the Colon, Rectum, and Anus. Philadelphia, W. B. Saunders, 1984, pp 384–396

19. McGarity WC: Colostomy: To irrigate or not to irrigate. J Med Assoc Ga, March 1973, p 93

20. Smith DB: Postoperative care of the patient with a colostomy or ileostomy. Am J Nurs 85(11):1246–1249, 1985

21. Smith DB, Johnson DE: Stoma complications. J Enterostom Ther 11(1):35–39, 1984

22. Sparberg M: To irrigate or not to irrigate. Ostomy Quarterly 7(3):46, 1970

23. Spratt JS: Special problems associated with colorectal and anal cancers, in Spratt JS (Ed): Neoplasms of the Colon, Rectum, and Anus. Philadelphia, W. B. Saunders, 1984, pp 329–407

24. Terranova O, Sander F, Rebuffat C, et al: Irrigation versus natural evacuation of left colostomy: A comparative study of 340 patients. Dis Colon Rectum 22:31–34, 1979

25. Turnbull RB, Gill N: Recent advances in colostomy surgery and care. Ostomy Quarterly 10(4):42–43, 1973

26. Warren R, McKittrick LS: Ileostomy for ulcerative colitis: Technique, complications, and management. Surg Gynecol Obstet 93:555–567, 1951

27. Watt RC: Colostomy irrigation: Yes or no. Am J Nurs 77:442–444, 1977

Dorothy B. Smith

# 4

# Multiple Stomas, Fistulas, and Draining Wounds

Cancer, by its very malignant characteristics, can push into, obstruct, invade, or perforate its neighboring tissues. It respects no boundaries locally and can affect more than one organ at a time. This activity may require the surgical construction of multiple stomas and the insertion of wound catheters and drains; it may also cause the development of spontaneous fistulas. Caring for patients with multiple openings can be exasperating. However, the goals of odor control, skin protection, drainage containment, infection control, and patient comfort can be combined and attained through effective pouch selection and application. In this pictorial chapter we present a variety of situations and suggest how to manage them by pouching. The reader interested in more information should consult the references and the readings listed in Appendix 4-1.

## MULTIPLE STOMAS

Multiple stomas may be planned as part of one procedure or may be created during subsequent operations.

### Stomas Created Concurrently

A total pelvic exenteration is an example of a planned procedure that includes a urinary diversion and a colostomy (Fig. 4-1). In women, it involves removing the bladder, rectum, ovaries, uterus, and possibly the vagina; in men, the bladder, rectum, prostate, and seminal vesicles are removed. The most common malignant indication for a pelvic exenteration is carcinoma of the cervix recurrent after definitive radiotherapy. The cervical tumor, sandwiched between the bladder and the rectum, extends locally anteriorly, posteriorly, or in both directions. To secure adequate surgical margins, the surgeon must remove the bladder and the rectum. Other indications for pelvic exenteration include cancer of the colon invading anteriorly into the bladder, cancer of the ovary, or a pelvic sarcoma such as rhabdomyosarcoma or leiomyosarcoma.

Because total pelvic exenteration is such an immense procedure and requires optimum patient and medical conditions for recovery, it is usually performed only as definitive treatment and not for palliation. When a patient is being evaluated for a pelvic exenteration, the health care team needs to consider carefully all of the preoperative, intraoperative, and postoperative factors discussed earlier for patients undergoing either a urinary or bowel diversion.

Preoperative stoma site selection and optimum surgical technique are extremely important so as to minimize the postoperative difficulties in caring for the ostomies. The operation has a tremendous physiologic and emotional effect on patients, and as a result their physical and mental reserves for learning may be low. The therapist takes this into consideration and teaches the care of one ostomy at a time. We have found

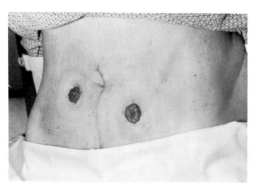

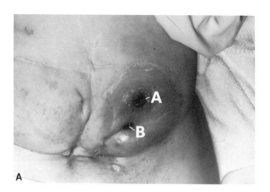

**Figure 4-1.** After a total exenteration, the urinary stoma is located slightly higher than the colostomy stoma.

rotation to be a good teaching method: a lesson in urostomy care one day, colostomy care the next day, and so on, emphasizing similarities along the way (see Chapter 5). If the patient intends to irrigate the colostomy, we wait until he returns for a follow-up visit to begin teaching

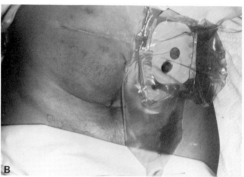

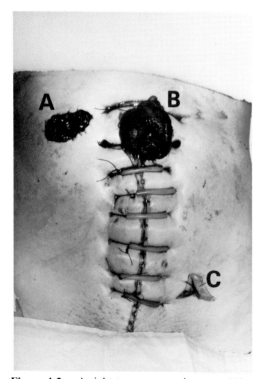

**Figure 4-3.** **A**, this patient has a descending colostomy (*A*) and a mucous fistula located inferiorly (*B*). The patient developed a fistula between her bladder and her mucous fistula bowel segment, draining urine out her mucous fistula. **B**, the same patient is wearing two pouches, a disposable urinary pouch over the mucous fistula and an overlapping colostomy pouch on the descending colostomy. The opening of the colostomy pouch has been cut off-center because the two stomas are so close. (Reprinted with permission from J Enterostom Ther 9[6]:61, 1982.[3])

**Figure 4-2.** A right transverse colostomy (*A*), a mucous fistula in the incision (*B*), and a Penrose drain (*C*) on the left.

the technique. At that time the patient has more strength and less discomfort from the perineal wound and also has had time to develop confidence and skill in emptying and changing both appliances. We have learned that if we try to teach everything at once, we increase the potential for failure and frustration. It is easier to prevent bad experiences than to help the patient recover lost confidence.

After a total pelvic exenteration, patients can recover fully and resume their daily social, work, family, and recreational activities. Pa-

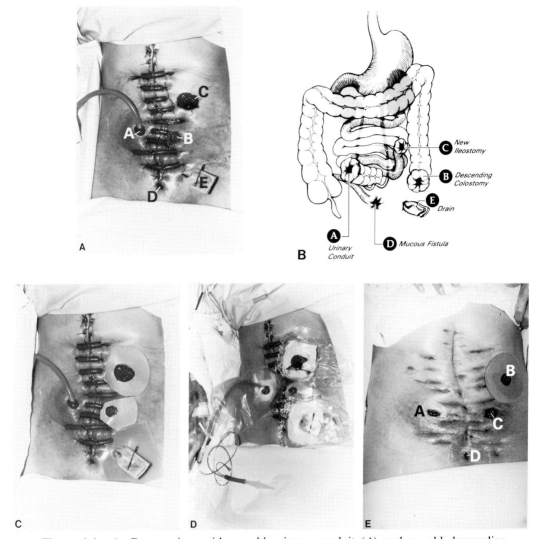

**Figure 4-4. A, B,** a patient with an old urinary conduit (*A*) and an old descending colostomy (*B*) required a new ileostomy (*C*), an incisional mucous fistula (*D*), and a Penrose drain (*E*) due to radiation injury to the bowel. **C,** skin barriers are applied to the ostomy and drain sites; note that the barriers have been cut away from the retention sutures. **D,** drainable pouches are applied over the skin barriers. **E,** the results after the incision has healed. The patient has a functioning conduit (*A*) and ileostomy (*B*), a nonfunctioning colostomy (*C*), and a mucous fistula (*D*). (**E** reprinted with permission from Cancer Bull 33:10, 1981.[1])

tients must maintain confidence in rehabilitation, and those providing their integrated care must aim for complete recovery.

Two stomas are also required when a colostomy or an ileostomy is combined with a mucous fistula (Fig. 4-2). Placement of both stomas should be considered carefully, since each may require a pouch. A section of bowel vented as a mucous fistula may become part of an enterofistula and provide bowel or urinary drainage (Fig. 4-3). Intestine, even though isolated from the functioning bowel, secretes mucus. If

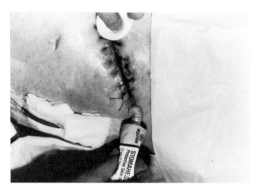

**Figure 4-5.** Paste is applied at the edges of an incisional fistula to make it smooth enough to hold a skin barrier and pouch securely.

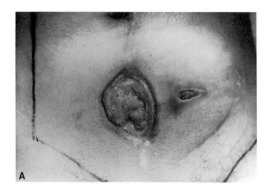

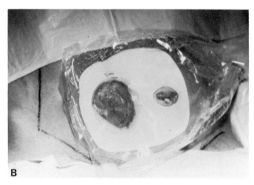

**Figure 4-6.** **A,** a tumor that has eroded through the skin and is draining at two sites. **B,** one appliance incorporates both drain sites. The openings are cut to match the drain sites, protecting the skin surface between the two sites. (Reprinted with permission from J Enterostom Ther 11[3]:120, 1984.[4])

the bowel has been irradiated, mucositis may occur, resulting in a clear liquid drainage that requires a pouch.

### Stomas Created at Different Times

In some instances, a patient may have a colostomy or ileostomy and a urinary diversion without undergoing a total pelvic exenteration. The ostomies may not even have been created for the same disease or at the same time. For example, a patient may have an ileostomy for benign disease and later require a urinary diversion for malignant disease. Or a patient may require one type of stoma as a primary component of cancer treatment and later require another type as a result of additional treatment, such as bowel or bladder damage from radiation (Fig. 4-4). The variables are numerous.

Physicians, nurses, and other members of the health care team must not make the mistake of assuming that, when a patient has one stoma, a second stoma will not affect him further. Each situation is different. A man with one stoma who has developed confidence in his care and has accepted the ostomy may receive a second stoma very matter-of-factly. Conversely, a woman who has had multiple negative experiences or who has never dealt with her feelings about her first ostomy may perceive a second ostomy as an unsurmountable tragedy. The second stoma may revive unresolved emotions from the first stoma, compounding the patient's reaction. Anyone working with these patients

must pay attention to the messages they send and provide at least the support they would receive if they were new patients.

### FISTULAS

A fistula is usually a spontaneous opening between two internal structures or between an internal organ and the skin. The type of drainage depends on the organ or structures involved. Fistulas may occur in many areas of the body, including the abdomen, thorax, pelvis, back, and neck. Because they are spontaneous, they frequently are located in difficult-to-treat places, adding to the challenge of applying a pouch. However, pouching a fistula has many advantages over monitoring it with multiple dressing

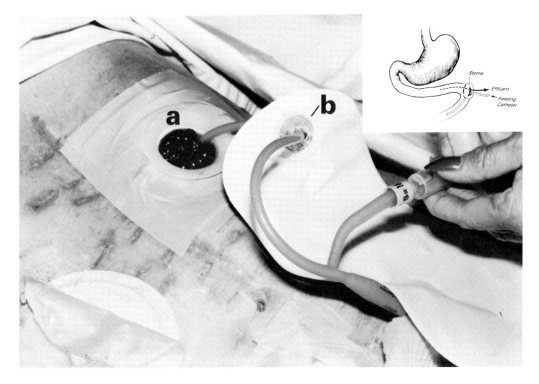

**Figure 4-7.** A loop jejunostomy. The proximal limb functions and the distal limb has a catheter inserted into it for feedings. A reusable faceplate (*a*) is applied around the stoma with a pouch to collect the jejunal drainage. The feeding catheter is brought out through the gas release valve (*b*) of an ileostomy pouch. The catheter is plugged when not used for feeding.

changes, including more effective drainage containment, skin protection, and odor control, greater ease and accuracy of output monitoring, more patient comfort, and reduced cost of supplies. Gauze dressing soon becomes soaked with the drainage, irritating the skin and requiring numerous dressing changes throughout the day.

As soon as a fistula is recognized, the skin around it should be protected with a barrier. An adhesive-backed, drainable, odor-resistant pouch should be selected, the model determined by the size and location of the fistula and the type of drainage. Fairly liquid drainage with little odor may be managed with one of the postoperative urinary pouches. These are the easiest to drain, but are usually not as odor resistant as bowel pouches. Available pouches include those that are sterile, those with connecting devices for straight drainage if the output is high, and those with a window opening

that is reclosable if wound inspection, packing, irrigations, or drain advancements are required.

The surrounding skin should be prepared in the same way as skin around a planned stoma. The area should be cleansed with warm water and dried thoroughly. If *Monilia* is present, it should be treated with Mycostatin powder and the powder covered with a plasticized dressing or surgical cement. If the fistula is in an incision or old scar or has irregular edges, one of the paste barriers may need to be applied as a filler. Paste can be applied around the edges of the fistula or in indented areas (Fig. 4-5). Only a small amount of paste is needed, and it should set a few seconds before the wafer and pouch are applied.

Figures 4-6 through 4-13 illustrate various fistulas and present examples of how they can be managed. The patient in Figure 4-6 had a pelvic sarcoma that eroded through the surface of the

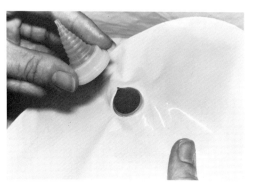

**Figure 4-8.** A commercially available access port that can be set into the pouch to support a catheter or tube. (Reprinted with permission from J Enterostom Ther 11[3]:116, 1984.[4])

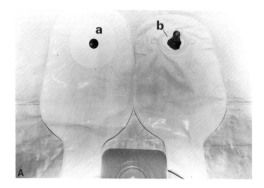

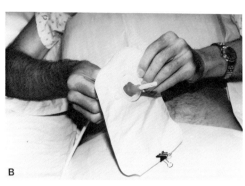

**Figure 4-9. A,** another method of preparing a pouch for a feeding tube is by placing a baby nipple through the pouch. A double-faced adhesive disc is placed on the outer (*a*) and inner (*b*) sides of the pouch to support the nipple. **B,** a feeding catheter is inserted through the nipple on the pouch, which is then attached over the stoma. The nipple fits snugly into the ostomy and acts as a dam to prevent reflux of the feeding.

skin. He was receiving external radiotherapy to the area as indicated by the skin markings. The drainage smelled foul. We applied a barrier paste as a thin ring around both areas to protect the skin edges and provide a more secure seal. We then cut one 8 × 8 inch wafer skin barrier and one large drainable fistula pouch to incorporate both sites. The openings were cut to the size of the drain sites to protect the skin. For this purpose, one may make precise patterns by tracing irregular or multiple openings onto a clear plastic or Saran wrapper such as is found on the packaging of skin barriers. One can place the pattern on the back side of the adhesive and cut on the tracings. The paper backing that is pulled off becomes a new pattern for the next pouch change.

The patient in Figure 4-7 had Gardner's syndrome, producing multiple gastrointestinal polyps. A loop jejunostomy was constructed and a feeding tube inserted into the distal loop. We applied a $1\frac{1}{2}$-inch Universal faceplate with a double-faced adhesive disc and skin-barrier wafer. We framed the plate with waterproof adhesive tape and applied a drainable reusable ileostomy pouch with a built-in gas-release valve, bringing the feeding catheter out through the gas-release valve. Another alternative for such a patient is to use a commercially available plastic access port through which to bring the catheter (Fig. 4-8). A third alternative for inserting a feeding catheter is shown in Figure 4-9. We used a two-piece drainable pouch, cutting the wafer to fit the stoma. We prepared the pouch by

inserting a baby nipple through an opening in the back. A double-faced adhesive disc stabilized the nipple on both sides. The catheter was inserted through the nipple as needed for feedings.

The patient in Figure 4-10 had a parastomal hernia repaired at the site of the sigmoid colostomy stoma. The parastomal incision was left open and a Penrose drain was placed lateral to the stoma site (Fig. 4-10*A*). To protect the open incision from stool contents, we formed a bridge with karaya paste at the stomal-incisional juncture. We cut a skin barrier wafer as a small washer, packed the wound with gauze strips, and applied a small drainable pouch over the

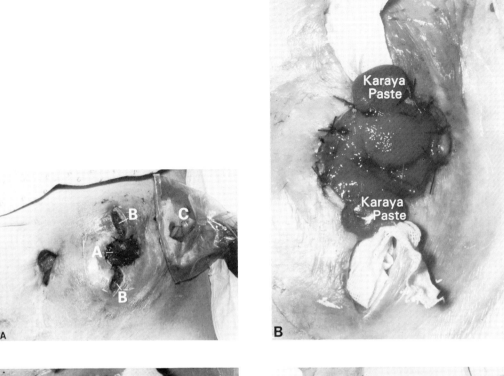

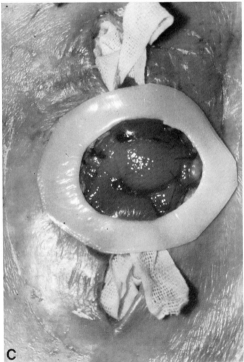

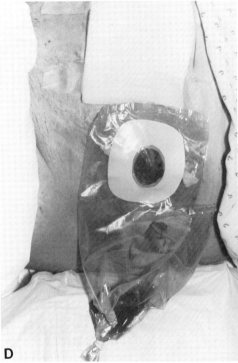

**Figure 4-10.** **A**, a patient with a sigmoid colostomy (*A*) developed a parastomal hernia. The hernia was repaired through two incisions left open to heal by secondary intention (*B*). A Penrose drain is shown with a pouch in place (*C*). **B**, the open incisions were packed with gauze. A small amount of karaya paste was used to bridge the areas connecting the incisions to the stoma; **C**, a small washer of a skin barrier wafer was applied over the paste; and **D**, a pediatric drain pouch was applied over the skin barrier. The appliance was removed daily so the incisions could be cleaned and repacked.

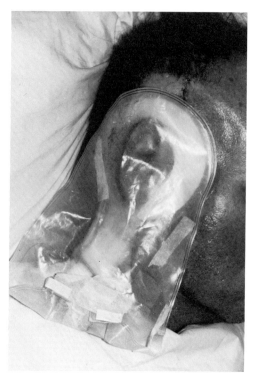

**Figure 4-11.** A skin barrier and pouch applied to a patient who has a cerebrospinal fluid leak through his ear. (Reprinted with permission from J Enterostom Ther 9[5]:20, 1982.[2])

colostomy and the Penrose drain site. We removed the pouch daily to care for the incision.

Not all fistulas are on the abdomen. They may occur on the head or neck, as illustrated in Figures 4-11 through 4-13.

Figure 4-11 illustrates a patient whose cerebrospinal fluid was leaking through a fistula tract in his ear. We applied a skin barrier and drainable pouch over the ear to collect the drainage and monitor the output.

The patient in Figure 4-12 had a colon interposition for esophageal cancer and developed a cervical fistula that drained saliva as well as regurgitated stomach contents. We painted surgical cement thinly around the fistula, spread a small amount of paste at either end of the opening, and applied the skin barrier and a flexible drainable pouch. This fistula had originally been managed by a catheter inserted in the wound and connected to suction, which had

restricted the patient's activity and delayed his discharge.

Figure 4-13 shows a postlaryngectomy patient who developed a cervical fistula very close to her tracheostomy. After filling the crevices with small amounts of paste and coating the area with surgical cement, we covered the tracheostomy and the fistula with a skin barrier. We then applied a drainable pediatric pouch over the barrier.

## TUBES AND DRAINS

Tubes and drains are a part of many surgical procedures. They may remain in place for a few days or, when the site is infected, be required for an extended period of time. Managing these drains by pouching techniques can be cost-effective, time-saving, and skin-sparing. The next four patients present a variety of situations ranging from a simple Penrose drain to a catheterized "blow-hole" incisional ileostomy.

Figure 4-14 shows a patient with a Penrose drain in place immediately after surgery. Because the surgeon wanted to advance the drain periodically, we applied a sterile-windowed wound-drain pouch over a skin barrier. It should be noted that the window was closed, but not securely enough; leakage occurred through the lower edge of the window (Fig. 4-14). The windows must be clean, dry, and closed securely all the way around the tract.

Figure 4-15 depicts a patient with uterine cervical carcinoma who had a right transverse colostomy. She developed a small-bowel fistula, into which the physician inserted a tube. When pouching the fistula, we were careful not to remove the eschar covering and extend the fistula. We applied a bridge of barrier paste followed by a thin coat of surgical cement over the healthy skin and a Telfa dressing over the eschar area. We then applied a skin-barrier wafer and drainable pouch and brought the tube out through a tape-reinforced area of the pouch.

Figure 4-16 (page 84) shows a patient who has widespread ovarian carcinoma. Her bowel was obstructed and the mesentery shortened by tumor. It was necessary to construct an incisional "blow-hole" ileostomy fitted with a catheter. To stabilize the catheter we used an inverted baby nipple, placing karaya paste under the nipple rim for a seal. We then painted a thin

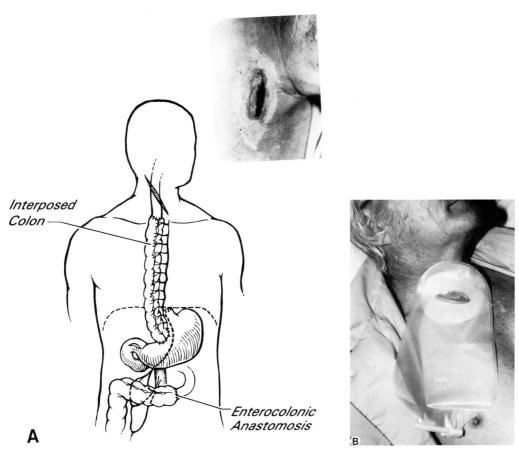

**Interposed Colon**

**Enterocolonic Anastomosis**

**A**

**B**

**Figure 4-12.** **A**, a fistula developed on a patient's neck after a colon interposition. Surgical cement was applied to the skin around the fistula; paste was used at both ends (inset). **B**, a drainable pouch and skin barrier have been applied over the neck fistula.

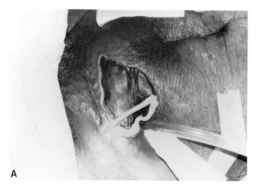

A

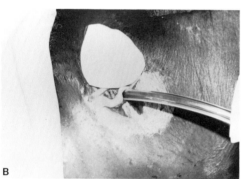

B

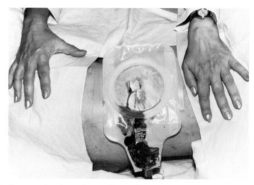

**Figure 4-14.** A patient immediately after abdominal surgery had a Penrose drain in place and a wound-drain pouch with an open window applied. The pouch is intact over the Penrose drain, but the window portal is leaking. The portal needs to be opened, cleaned with an alcohol wipe or gauze, dried, and then resealed.

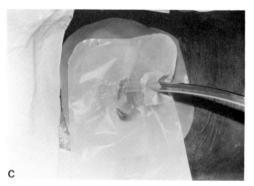

C

**Figure 4-13.** **A**, a patient with a cervical neck fistula (*A*) located near a tracheostomy. **B**, a skin barrier wafer, cut to encompass both stomas, is applied over surgical cement and paste. **C**, a pediatric pouch is applied over the neck fistula to prevent fistula drainage from spilling into the tracheostomy. (Reprinted with permission from J Enterostom Ther 9[5]:23, 1982.[2])

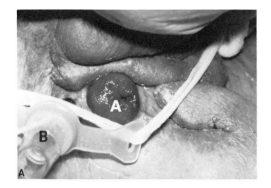

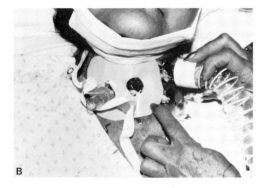

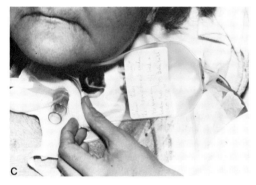

**Figure 4-15. A,** a small-bowel fistula that has developed in a patient with cervical cancer. A catheter is inserted directly into the fistula. A bridge of skin barrier paste is applied across the eschar that had developed over the wound. **B,** a thin coat of surgical cement is painted on the skin around the catheter and a Telfa dressing is cut and applied over the eschar. **C,** a skin barrier and pouch are applied over the wound. The catheter is brought out through the pouch and reinforced with tape.

coat of surgical cement on the skin and applied Telfa dressings over the open incision. We prepared a pouch with a reinforced area for the tube and covered the entire incision and pouch with a large skin-barrier wafer. We then brought a catheter through the pouch and anchored it with plastic tape. An access port would have been useful here to bring the catheter through; however, if no access port is available, the pouch can be reinforced with plastic tape, a piece of the skin-barrier wafer, or a double-faced adhesive before the opening is cut. If reinforcement is not used, the plastic of the pouch may split. After the catheter has been brought through the opening, plastic tape can be used to seal the opening and support the tube.

## CONCLUSION

Knowledge of the available pouches and accessories and creativity in selecting and applying the equipment are the keys to effectively managing most fistulas and draining wounds. These, along with multiple stomas, require patience and resourcefulness from the health care team. The originality required to manage these fistulas provides a challenge, but the reward for doing so—a comfortable patient—is well worth the effort.

## APPENDIX 4-1

### Suggested Readings

1. Dunavant MK: Wound and fistula management, in Broadwell D, Jackson B (Eds): Principles of Ostomy Management. St. Louis, C. V. Mosby, 1982, pp 658–686
2. Irrgang S, Bryant R: Management of the enterocutaneous fistula. J Enterstom Ther 11(6):211–225, 1984
3. Irving M, Beadle C: External intestinal fistulas: Nursing care and surgical procedures, in Brooke BN, Jeter KF, Todd TP (Eds): Stomas. Clin Gastroenterol 2:327–336, 1982

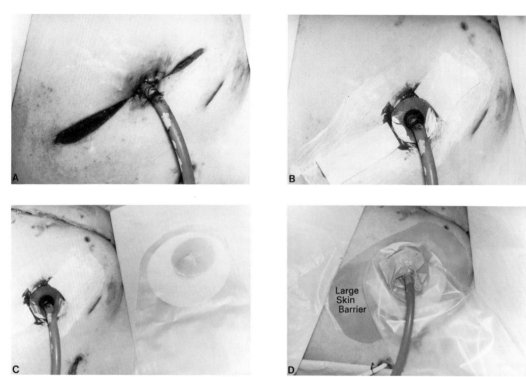

**Figure 4-16.** A patient with widespread ovarian cancer required a "blow-hole" ileostomy to relieve bowel obstruction. The bowel was matted with tumor and was not long enough to be used for stoma construction. **A,** a catheter is inserted through the skin incision into the bowel. **B,** the catheter in the blow-hole is stabilized by an inverted baby nipple. We spread karaya paste under the nipple rim as a sealant, painted surgical cement thinly on the skin, and placed Telfa dressings over the incisions. **C,** a drainable pouch is prepared. The opening for the tube is reinforced by a skin barrier wafer. **D,** the entire incisional area is covered with a large skin barrier. A pouch is applied over the barrier, and the tubing is brought through it and secured with tape. (**A** and **C** reprinted with permission from J Enterostom Ther 11[3]:120, 1984.[4])

## REFERENCES

1. Bates M: Fistulas and draining wounds. Cancer Bull 33:19–21, 1981
2. Rodriguez DB: Fistulas of the head and neck. J Enterostom Ther 9(5):20–24, 1982
3. Rodriguez DB: Stoma site selection. J Enterostom Ther 9(6):60–62, 1982
4. Smith DB: Abdominal fistulas. J Enterostom Ther 11(3):116–121, 1984

Dorothy B. Smith

# 5

# Patient Teaching

A 67-year-old accountant retired to Florida several years ago so that he and his wife could enjoy outdoor living. His life was rudely interrupted when he learned that he had bladder cancer, which required removing the bladder and constructing an ileal conduit. His postoperative convalescence was uneventful, but he was never taught how to manage his ostomy appliance independently and came to rely on his wife to change it for him. As a result, he has withdrawn from his twice-weekly golf foursome and remains at home, fearful to venture far without his wife at his side. The possibility of the ostomy's leaking when help is not available is a constant, nagging fear. He has become depressed, irritable, and preoccupied with somatic complaints.

This scenario is acted out all too frequently under different guises by cancer patients with ostomies. The problem is basically one of dependency. We should never forget that a person cannot accept an ostomy if he does not feel confident in caring for it himself. Someone who depends on another for ostomy care has a handicap far greater than the physical burden of the ostomy.

It is axiomatic that rehabilitation cannot occur without independence, and independence requires patient learning. It follows, then, that careful teaching is an important prerequisite to a patient's independence and rehabilitation.

Effective patient teaching begins preoperatively when the patient and family first learn about the need for an ostomy. It is founded on the early interpersonal relationships that form between the patient and the members of the health care team, relationships that are vital to the learner-teacher interaction that will follow surgery. This relationship should be constructive, not dependent, and should grow organically as the patient progresses from the acute recovery period to convalescence to self-care.

Although in this chapter the focus is on teaching the *patient*, emphasizing independence through learning, we do not exclude the *family*; patient and family are considered together as a unit: the learners. The teaching principles apply equally to both.

## PRINCIPLES OF TEACHING

Teaching is a function that cannot be left to chance. Although all members of the health care team share the responsibility of seeing that patients are taught self-care, good teachers know that one person must be responsible for the process—for assessment, planning, lessons, return demonstrations, and follow-through. This person should keep accurate patient-teaching records so that all members of the team can be kept advised of the patient's specific learning needs, any barriers that impede learning, and the progress made in the lessons toward self-care.

Learning seldom takes place unless the learner engages in some activity, preferably both mental and physical. Nowhere is this principle stated more clearly than: "*When I hear it, I forget it. When I see it, I remember it. When I do it, I know it.*" Learning is never passive. Fre-

THE CANCER PATIENT WITH AN OSTOMY
ISBN 0-8089-1807-9

quently we see patients who, because of their professional or social standings, try to intimidate the teacher by refusing to practice their own ostomy care. We do not allow that! We apply the same principles of teaching to all patients and insist that they practice their care under supervision. Otherwise, the results can be tragic.

Everyone involved in caring for patients with ostomies should expect that they will take over their own care. Patients usually readily accept this goal at the outset, but their confidence must be continually reinforced, especially by their physicians and nurses, if they are to achieve complete independence.

"Demonstration–return demonstration" is a very effective method for teaching self-care to patients with ostomies. No one should expect them to learn their complete care after a single lesson. An all-too-common mistake made by hospital personnel is to expect that patients can learn to care for themselves on the day of discharge. Trying to learn the entire procedure in a hurried manner just before going home leaves an already vulnerable patient open to failure and frustration. An even greater error is to expect a visiting nurse or home-care nurse to give a patient the first lesson in self-care after he has been discharged from the hospital.

Instead, we must provide ample time, while patients are recovering from surgery, for demonstration and supervised practice. This way, by the time they go home their ostomy care is something they feel confident about performing, not just something they have read about or watched someone else do. To develop confidence while in the hospital, patients should have to struggle with frustrations, experience failure, and enjoy success. They should have time to encounter a variety of situations and to find methods of care suitable to their capabilities. Only then are they really ready to care for their ostomy at home.

## FACTORS AFFECTING LEARNING

A person who has a newly created ostomy is projected simultaneously into two roles: that of patient and that of learner. Often the demands of one interfere with the needs of the other. Such external factors as physician orders, nurse staffing, bed use, hospital schedule, or teacher's obligations can override the patient's learning needs. Although the external factors cannot be ignored, the teacher should attempt to match teaching time and technique to the learner's needs.

A number of individual factors affect each learner's ability to respond to the teacher. Although these factors can be examined independently, the health care team should be cautious about categorizing patients according to group traits. We must provide all patients the opportunity to try for themselves, to learn what they can, and to achieve independence on their own terms.

### Physical Factors

*Illness*

A patient's ability to participate in the learning process is influenced greatly by his illness. Through no choice of his own, he is a patient first, a learner second. Patients usually find it very difficult to focus attention on learning something new when they are multiply distracted by pain, fever, nausea, tubes, and any of the other assaults that follow surgery. We have found that teaching is much more effective when it is begun preoperatively, before patients experience the pain or discomfort of their incisions, the nasogastric tubes, the intravenous lines, or the catheters or have to spend all their energy in coughing, turning, and ambulating. In addition, medications that control pain, nausea, or other symptoms may erase memory; when this happens, efforts to teach patients are wasted. It is imperative, therefore, that before beginning any instruction, either preoperatively or postoperatively, the teacher evaluate the patient's level of comfort and medication.

*Age*

Age is a factor that influences learning, not only for those at the extremes, but also for those in the middle years.

*Youth.* Because a child moves rapidly through a number of distinct developmental stages that involve particular developmental tasks, he can best be reached through things that he has already experienced.[3] Cartoons, puppets, coloring books, stickers, dolls, stuffed animals, and other toys are useful tools for teaching children. A preschooler who, as an infant, has undergone a total pelvic exenteration resulting in a urinary diversion and a colostomy may learn some of her ostomy care by cutting out and applying minipouches on a doll. Decorating her colostomy irrigation equipment with stickers and colorful flowers may do much to allay her fears and allow her to become interested in all that is going on around her.[7]

Children are surprisingly open and receptive to learning.[5] They want to find out how things work and to gain control over themselves; they want to do what they see others doing. Because children are naturally curious, the best teaching is a response to this curiosity. We begin by letting them play with the equipment and practice using it while there is no threat of failure. We then make sure that the first tasks we pose are ones they can perform. If they begin with a failure, they may not have enough confidence to try again. (For more information, see Chapter 11, "Special Problems in Children.")

*Adulthood.* Even more subtle factors can influence an adult's ability to learn. By adulthood, people usually have developed independence and defined a role, such as breadwinner, homemaker, parent, husband, or wife. Inevitably, illness and hospitalization impose a degree of dependency, thus altering a patient's accepted role. To counteract this unfamiliar situation and to assert their independence, adults who feel they are being treated like children may resist learning.

Patients with a new ostomy frequently ask the person caring for the stoma, "How can you stand to do this all the time?" referring to cleaning the skin of feces or urine. The nurse must not make the error of responding with a remark that compares the adult to a child. "It's no different from caring for babies" or "We clean up babies" is not an encouraging reply. The patient already has a low self-image and needs a positive statement from the nurse. A more acceptable reply may be, "Why should I be bothered? Urine and stool are natural parts of every healthy person." One could continue with something like this: "Perhaps you are concerned because, in our culture, we have taught ourselves to be embarrassed by elimination." Another possible response could be: "The doctor has diverted your stool (or urine) to your abdomen to help you function normally. You're no

different from before, except that the opening for your elimination has been moved." Replying with a statement in this vein, spoken matter-of-factly and in a supportive manner, minimizes the patient's embarrassment and does not imply that he is childlike.

Showing respect and regard for a patient as an adult is exceptionally important when teaching something as personal and private as ostomy care. Not only does caring for the ostomy involve learning a new skill—a new technique of private hygiene—but it also arouses deeply subjective emotions about relearning continence. In our culture, acquiring continence of stool and urine is a very hard-learned, emotionally charged developmental task.

In teaching adults, we work to establish a climate of mutual respect. We keep interactions friendly and informal, allowing the learners to participate in defining their own needs for learning.[2] Patients are more willing to learn and to be active in performing their own care if they recognize that what they are learning has immediate and direct applicability to their lives: they can resolve an identified problem, that of appliance leakage, if they learn to care for their ostomy.

*Old age.* Aging itself, unless accompanied by disease, has little affect on one's ability to learn—only on the rate of learning.[1] Disease, however, can chronically erode memory, and medication, surgery, or unfamiliar surroundings can impair memory temporarily. Postoperative confusion and lack of mental alertness frequently follow a long and stressful operation in an elderly patient. When this occurs, it is wise to delay teaching, allowing the patient extra time after surgery to "wake up."

The teacher should plan to give elderly people special considerations. Frequently, they are strongly motivated to remain independent and are eager to learn self-care, if only the teacher can allot them extra time and patience. A sensitive teacher allows for reduced learning speed or for problems with diminished sensory or motor capabilities. We have learned to use repetition, to label the equipment according to the steps of care, and to avoid any actions or mannerisms that make the patient feel hurried. Pressure only increases patients' frustration and decreases their motivation to try.

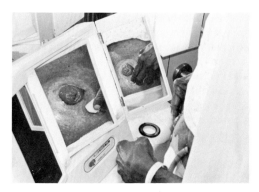

**Figure 5-1.** A patient with impaired vision may find that using a lighted magnifying mirror helps in stomal care.

*Dexterity*

Caring for an ostomy and applying an appliance require some degree of manual dexterity. People with an intentional tremor, arthritis, a disabled arm, or an extremity weakness may need to have the equipment and the care routine modified to match their capabilities. The health care team must focus on the goal—independence—and remember that it can be achieved in more than one way.

Nurses who assess patients with impaired dexterity learn to share their concerns with the patients. Frequently patients can provide the solution. From experience, they may already be adept at compensating for their diminished dexterity and not need special care at all. For example, when a woman with arthritis or an intentional tremor says that she quilts at home, she implies that she is quite capable of mastering manual tasks. The alert teacher lets patients tell—or, better still, show—what they can do.

*Vision*

Visual aids, such as a lighted magnifying mirror, may help patients with impaired vision to see the stoma (Fig. 5-1). Those with minimal vision, or none at all, can learn to do their own care by touch. The teacher should make every effort to help visually impaired patients learn to care for themselves so that they can remain independent.

**Education**

Prior education is not a measure of a person's intelligence or ability to learn. A "well-educated" person does not necessarily learn more, faster, or better than a person less educated. However, the amount of formal education may affect a person's skill in ostomy care in unexpected ways.

Illness, anxiety, attitude, or other factors can completely incapacitate a highly educated person and a less-educated person alike. However, patients with little formal education may be accustomed to compensating by exerting extra effort to learn and may be highly motivated by pride to learn their care. Such patients may also be very adept at thinking with their hands, using their imaginations to make parts fit or an appliance work. Conversely, intellectually oriented patients may have had very little experience using their hands for manual tasks or reasoning with mechanical devices. Their success and confidence have resulted from mental efforts, and they may be frightened at the thought of having to control an appliance.

**Attitudinal Factors**

*Motivation*

Patients' attitudes can powerfully influence their ability to learn. First, patients must want to learn, and second, they must believe that what they are asked to learn is important to them. This is especially true for patients who have just experienced life-threatening surgery and are concentrating on survival. At this stage it is difficult to be motivated to learn about future self-care.[1]

Patients develop their own attitudes from internal sources, yet respond to and are influenced by the attitudes of their physicians, members of the hospital staff, their families, and other patients. Attitude is contagious.[4]

This fact should be employed consciously in teaching. When a teacher's attitude is positive, showing confidence in a patient's ability to learn, the patient senses it. The teacher, however, must be sincere, since patients quickly detect faked responses and interpret them as doubt.

Molding attitudes occupies a large part of the time the teacher spends with a patient and family. The teacher recognizes that the learner's best work may never equal the teacher's second-best and therefore never attempts comparisons. Instead, the teacher rewards any effort or attempt, even though the actual task may need much improvement. If patients feel their efforts have not been successful, or good enough, their motivation to try again decreases. If, however, they feel that they are making progress toward a satisfactory outcome, they remain motivated to continue learning. Therefore the effective teacher provides the learner with specific feedback and positive reinforcement during the process.

Attitude and motivation fluctuate throughout learning. If a patient's attitude is negative and he resists the teacher's efforts, the physician should be prepared to step in. The physician must remind the patient that doctor, nurse, and patient are part of the same health care team, that he supports what the nurse is doing, and that he will not discharge any patient who is unable to perform his ostomy care. These words may sound harsh at the time, but frequently they are what are needed to encourage a patient out of apathy.

*Anxiety*

People who have cancer are bound to react emotionally to their illness. If they also have a new ostomy, they quite naturally are emotionally upset by their altered body and the change in their routine of personal hygiene. Patients are anxious about their cancer and the treatment, about pain, about whether their spouse will still love them, whether they can return to work, and whether they will be able to care for their ostomy. Anxiety can be a great deterrent to learning, markedly affecting its quality and pace.

Anxiety is manifested in several ways. It can occur as anger, depression, humor, sarcasm, doubt, or dependency.[6] Whatever the symptom, it must alert the teacher to the presence of anxiety. Helping the patient and family resolve their fears and overcome their anxiety may be the first constructive step the teacher can take.

*Trust*

Patient learning is influenced by the level of trust and rapport that exists between teacher and learner. If patients do not know or trust their teachers, a significant amount of learning may not occur. Nurses can begin to encourage trust in the early postoperative period while physically caring for the stoma. They can use this time to build confidence while providing physical care—changing the appliance for the patient

skillfully and without causing discomfort or pain. This trust then transfers automatically as the nurse becomes the teacher.

## TEACHING PLAN

The first few postoperative lessons in ostomy care take place while the patient is lying in bed. At first the nurse changes the appliance gently, quickly, and without confusion, but while doing so she talks to the patient. If appropriate, she can explain what she is doing and try to demonstrate to the patient and interested family members the basic techniques involved. She should answer any questions without becoming too technical in her replies.

At the next appliance change, the nurse should try to get the patient involved. She should show the appliance to the patient and explain how to prepare and apply it. As she removes the old appliance and cleans the skin, she can continue to explain the technique. Remember, repetition is important in learning, especially for patients who are taking mind-altering medications, having their sleep disrupted, and suffering multiple sensory assaults. While the appliance is off, the patient should be shown the stoma and encouraged to touch it and observe its features.

During the third appliance change patients can usually be cajoled to take a more active role. They can help to trace a pattern on the pouch and to cut the opening. They can remove the old appliance and check the condition of the stoma. The nurse once again describes the necessary steps in cleansing the skin. As patients become involved more and more in the learning process, they should be encouraged to practice each part until they have mastered the whole.

By the fourth or fifth appliance change, patients are usually able to prepare a new pouch, remove the old pouch, cleanse the skin, and apply the new pouch. Not all patients can learn at this pace, of course; some move more quickly and others need more repetition and practice.

As patients progress, the nurse should stress the need for them to integrate home ostomy care into their usual personal hygiene routine. Patients should begin to think about how they will arrange the equipment at home. We have found that, when space and conditions permit, most patients prefer to prepare the new pouch in the bathroom, placing it on the wash-bowl counter. They can then remove the old pouch at the wash bowl, using warm water and a washcloth to push the skin gently away from the adhesive of the pouch. In the tub or shower they can cleanse the stoma and surrounding skin with mild soap and a washcloth. The area should be rinsed thoroughly and then patted dry with an absorbent towel. At this point, a patient is ready to apply the new pouch.

In preparing patients for home care it is important that the teacher be aware of the home situation. We are quickly reminded of a patient we instructed, employing guidelines similar to those described above, only to become cha-grined months later when we learned that he had no indoor plumbing!

Once patients have had a chance to practice under the teacher's supervision and have visu-alized the steps involved, we have found it helpful to provide them with written instructions (see Appendices 5-1 through 5-6). Of course written instructions should never replace dem-onstrations and practice, but they are useful reminders for patients, both in the hospital and, later, at home.

## CONCLUSION

Teaching a cancer patient with an ostomy involves interaction between the teacher and the learner, based on the learner's needs. It requires a specific investment of time from one member of the health care team, who assumes the re-sponsibility of assessing the patient's needs and capabilities, planning the lessons, demonstrating the care, supervising the patient during practice, and evaluating what the patient has learned. Every member of the health care team partici-pates in this process in some way, either through supportive encouragement, actual demonstra-tion while performing ostomy care, supervision while the patient practices, answering questions, or allaying fears.

The goal of teaching a patient with an ostomy is independence in care and a return to normal activities. The task of applying an ostomy pouch is not difficult, but if the process becomes colored with emotions, pain, mental barriers, and physical limitations it can grow into an overwhelming responsibility. Successful teaching is measured in patient and family learn-ing.

## APPENDIX 5-1

### How to Apply a Skin Barrier and Temporary Pouch

A.  Prepare the pouch.
   1.  Trace a pattern on the white side of the skin barrier.
   2.  Cut out the pattern.
   3.  Cut the backing on the pouch to match the pattern.
   4.  Remove the adhesive back of the pouch.
   5.  Put deodorant soap and lemon spray in a colostomy pouch.
   6.  Stick the pouch to the skin barrier.
   7.  Remove the adhesive backing from the skin barrier.
B.  Prepare the skin.
   1.  Remove the old pouch from the skin. Use warm water on a washcloth and gently push the skin away from the pouch.
   2.  Wash the skin and stoma with warm water.
   3.  Dry the skin well.
   4.  Apply a thin ring of skin barrier paste directly around the stoma, if needed. Allow the paste to dry long enough so that it does not pull away when touched.
C.  Care for the skin if it is red.
   1.  Dust Mycostatin powder on the skin. Wipe off excess.
   2.  Pat Skin Prep or a similar wipe on the skin. Let it dry.
D.  Apply the pouch.
E.  "Picture frame" the pouch with four short strips of waterproof adhesive tape.

## APPENDIX 5-2

### How to Apply a Reusable Urinary Appliance Using an Adhesive Disc

1.  Remove the faceplate with warm water on gauze or a washcloth.
2.  Wash the stoma and the area around the stoma with warm water. Rinse well and dry.
3.  Measure the stoma. Select a faceplate $\frac{1}{16}$-inch larger than the stoma.

4. Place the faceplate on the adhesive disc and trace a pattern of the opening onto the disc with a pencil.
5. Cut out the opening traced.
6. Place the faceplate on a flat surface. Remove the release paper from the disc and press the disc to the faceplate by smoothing the surface with the fingertips.
7. Remove the release paper from the back side of the disc and place it to one side.
8. Hold a wick to the stoma or urine opening by rolling a piece of gauze or holding a tampon to the opening while the skin is drying.
9. Center the opening of the faceplate over the stoma. Be sure that the belt hooks are pointed straight across the body.
10. Press the faceplate to the skin and hold it in place for a few seconds.
11. Attach a belt if needed. Make it snug but not tight.
12. "Picture frame" the faceplate with four short strips of tape.
13. Stretch the opening of the pouch over the lip and the raised part of the faceplate, beginning at the bottom of the faceplate.
14. Place the Bead "O" Ring (elastic) on the pouch; begin at the bottom and pull it up over the pouch. Secure the elastic by sliding the bead down toward the pouch.
15. Close the outlet valve at the bottom of the pouch.
16. Remove the pouch daily or every second day, as preferred, to rinse out or inspect the stoma.
17. Remove the faceplate every six to seven days and thoroughly clean the skin and stoma.

## APPENDIX 5-3

### How to Apply a Reusable Urinary Appliance Using Cement

1. Remove the faceplate with warm water on gauze or a washcloth.
2. Wash the stoma and surrounding area with warm water. Rinse well.
3. Dry the skin thoroughly (moisture on the skin keeps the appliance from adhering). Hold a wick to the stoma by rolling a piece of gauze or holding a tampon to the opening while the skin is drying.

4. Apply a thin, smooth coat of cement to the disc of the appliance and a thin coat to the skin. Allow each coat to dry a few seconds; the cement feels tacky when it is dry.
5. Apply the faceplate with the stoma exactly centered in the opening. (If the appliance touches the stoma it will rub and irritate it.)
6. "Picture frame" four strips of tape around the disc to hold it securely.
7. Put the belt on snugly but not too tightly.

## APPENDIX 5-4

### How to Apply an Ileostomy Pouch

1. Assemble all equipment: a clean pouch, skin barrier, washcloth or gauze squares.
2. Remove the old pouch with a warm, moist washcloth or gauze.
3. Wash the skin and stoma with warm water. Rinse well and dry.
4. Keep the skin dry by holding a gauze wick to the stoma to keep drainage off the skin.
5. Apply a thin ring of skin barrier paste directly around the stoma. Allow the paste to dry long enough so that it does not pull away when touched with a finger.
6. Apply a skin barrier washer to fit snugly around the stoma.
7. Apply the pouch with the stoma centered; press the adhesive to the skin to form a seal.
8. Secure the bottom of the pouch with a clamp or closure.

(Hints: (1) Empty the pouch frequently to avoid leaks. (2) Spray Periwash and deodorant into the pouch to help keep it clean and odor-free.)

## APPENDIX 5-5

### How to Apply an Ostomy Bag with a Karaya Ring

1. Gently remove the old appliance, using warm water on a 4" × 4" gauze or a cloth. If adhesive remains on the skin, gently roll it off with a finger.
2. Rinse the skin and dry it thoroughly.
3. Remove the adhesive backing from the pouch.

4. Position the pouch opening around the stoma to form a seal. (*Note*: The opening of a pouch with a karaya ring may touch the stoma; the karaya softens and melts and does not irritate the stoma.)
5. Press the adhesive around the stoma to form a seal.
6. Apply deodorant inside the pouch.
7. If desired, apply mineral oil or baby oil inside the clean pouch to keep stool from sticking to it, thus making it easier to clean.
8. Close the pouch at the bottom with a clamp or closure.
9. Empty the pouch as needed.
10. Clean and rinse the inside of the pouch at least once daily.

## APPENDIX 5-6

### How to Irrigate a Colostomy

*Technique*

1. Assemble all equipment: irrigation set, lubricant, washcloth, paper bag for the soiled pouch.
2. Put one quart of warm tap water in the irrigation container.
3. Expel the air from the tubing by letting water run through the tube.
4. Fasten the irrigation sleeve around the stoma with the bottom of the sleeve in the commode. Spray inside the sleeve with Periwash to reduce odor and facilitate cleaning the sleeve.
5. Lubricate the irrigation catheter or cone and gently insert it two to three inches while the water is running. Caution: the water is intended to stimulate the bowel

gently to evacuate. If the catheter is inserted too far or the irrigation bag held too high, the water goes high into the bowel and takes several hours to return.
6. If cramping occurs, clamp the tubing shut for a few seconds.
7. When all the water is in, remove the catheter or cone.
8. The irrigation may take 45 minutes to an hour to complete.
9. If the return flow is slow, massage the abdomen or stand up and move about, keeping the end of the sleeve clamped.
10. If no leakage occurs between irrigations, place a 4″ × 4″ gauze or stoma cap over the stoma.

*Advice*

1. Water should be warm, not hot or cold. Cold water may cause cramps and hot water may injure the bowel.
2. Keep the skin around the stoma clean by washing it daily with warm water. Shower or bathe without a dressing or pouch, if desired.
3. Eat any foods you ate before surgery.
4. Resume any activities you performed before surgery, after your doctor gives his or her permission.
5. Irrigate your colostomy daily at first, or as instructed before you leave the hospital. Later irrigate every other day if that was when your bowels normally moved.
6. Wash the equipment after use with mild soap and water.
7. The results from your irrigation will not be the same every day. Do not repeat the irrigation if results are poor on a given day; just wait and irrigate again the next day.

## REFERENCES

1. Bille DA: Barriers to the teaching-learning process, in Bille DA: Practical Approaches to Patient Teaching. Boston, Little, Brown, 1981, pp 69–84
2. Bille DA: Developing a philosophy of patient teaching, in Bille DA: Practical Approaches to Patient Teaching. Boston, Little, Brown, 1981, pp 27–34
3. Erikson E: Youth and the life cycle. Children 7:43–50, 1960
4. Frankl VE: Man's Search for Meaning. New York, Pocket Books, 1959
5. Holt J: How Children Learn. New York, Dell, 1967
6. Narrow BW: Selected aspects of instruction, in Narrow BW (Ed): Patient Teaching in Nursing Practice. New York, Wiley Medical Publishers, 1979, pp 166–180
7. Rodriguez DB: Teaching the preschooler with two ostomies. J Enterostom Ther 9(1):18–19, 1982

Susan Dudas

# 6

# Psychosocial Aspects of Patient Care

Today ostomies are created for people of all ages and for many reasons, including congenital anomalies, trauma, inflammatory bowel disease, and cancer. All of these patients have needs that are uniquely related to their type of surgery and to their age group, but those whose ostomy is a consequence of cancer have an additional set of special needs. This becomes vivid when one compares the reaction of a symptom-free patient who is informed that he has cancer and needs an ostomy with that of a patient with ulcerative colitis who has endured severely painful episodes for years and therefore views ostomy surgery hopefully, as a potential relief and cure. Cancer patients must deal not only with the proposed ostomy and all of its implications, but also with the new diagnosis of cancer and all of its implications. The resulting stress threatens their very psychological integrity.

Ostomy surgery results in loss of bowel or bladder control, abdominal disfigurement, and, at times, sexual dysfunction.[31,32] Cancer frequently is viewed as a dread and terminal disease associated with pain, other disabling symptoms, isolation, and death, even though a growing number of persons now survive. As patients confront the double realities of cancer and an ostomy, they suffer anger and confusion. Patients whose lives are threatened by disease feel helpless, out of control.[22] They fear that, after ostomy surgery for cancer, they will suffer rejection, shame, and disfigurement; their self-esteem is low; they have difficulty forming new relationships.[7,29]

Sontag,[26] in analyzing attitudes of society, has compared the stigma of cancer today to that of tuberculosis in the nineteenth century. Both are associated with "punitive and sentimental fantasies." She notes that these fantasies, mysteries, and myths become an additional burden to be carried by patients and families who are confronted not only with the diagnosis of cancer but also with its connotations of doom, punishment, and repression. Patients often vacillate between the fears associated with cancer —that it is contagious, that the disease progresses painfully, and that death is imminent—and their hope that their condition is surgically removable and curable.

Patients' responses to cancer are individual, reflecting their own personalities, self-images, cultures, and previous experiences. They can react with anxiety, depression, hostility, a sense of powerlessness, a feeling of hopelessness, or with a combination of these emotions.[16] Even though cure rates are much better today, a diagnosis of cancer continues to be devastating to patients and their families.

Patients with cancer are confronted, often for the first time, with the reality of their own mortality.[16] Weisman and Worden[34] found that patients frequently think about death during the first 100 days after hearing a diagnosis of cancer. When a patient requires ostomy surgery for cancer, these 100 days also include the emotional trauma of adjusting to a loss of body function, a change in body image, dependence on health professionals for learning ostomy care, and a multitude of other psychosocial and financial concerns. The threat of death, however, may overshadow the concerns about the ostomy at this time.

The patient who has cancer and an ostomy cannot suppress, deny, or "forget" the disease after surgery as readily as can a patient whose cancer has been removed with no visible anatomic or functional change. Instead, the diagnosis and threat of cancer are reinforced each time the patient sees or has to manage the ostomy. This constant reminder and reinforcement may be a major factor in the fear of a recurrence, a threat that may overwhelm some patients and their families. Even when surgery has been performed at an early stage and cure is expected, the patient with cancer is often uncertain about the future because of this fear. When the fear of recurrence is excessive, it can lead patients to a debilitating preoccupation with the disease.[24]

## ASSESSMENT

Each person copes with cancer and ostomy surgery in an individual way. What one manages easily can overwhelm another. Assessing the patient's strengths and limitations, therefore, is the first step in assisting a patient appropriately.

### Psychosocial Resources

It is necessary to determine the actual and potential resources available to facilitate the patient's rehabilitation. Therefore, in addition to obtaining information on the patient's current and past health status, health professionals must gather psychosocial data that can be used to predict the person's reaction to cancer and an ostomy and the future quality of his or her life.

A discussion about the patient's prior experience with people who had cancer or an ostomy helps the professional to assess the patient's level of knowledge and expectations, both positive and negative.[1] Other essential information includes: patients' perceptions of their situation; patients' usual coping strategies; available support systems (family, significant others, and community resources); patients' educational level; their occupation and employment status; the adequacy of their financial and insurance resources; their spiritual resources; and their religious affiliations and the significance of religion in their lives. Other items to assess when helping patients plan for their needs after discharge are the type of residence in which they live, the number and type of dependents and support persons in the home, the availability of resources for transportation, and available home-care services and self-help groups.

Identifying and, if possible, strengthening the support systems available to patients and their families are important components of the assessment. A patient may identify someone outside the nuclear family on whom he relies and who can be a resource in a crisis. However, the health professional must determine the actual availability of such a person, in case the patient has misinterpreted the relationship, the commitment, or the availability of this special support resource. Expanded information about support systems is particularly necessary when, for example, the person has traveled to a medical center distant from his home and family.

To establish realistic goals with patients, the health professional needs information about the usual life-style pattern of the patients and the changes anticipated as a result of the cancer and the ostomy. Information about sexuality is also an important part of the psychosocial assessment (see Chapter 7). To serve patients adequately, health professionals must recognize sexuality as an integral part of their psychosocial needs.

### The Older Patient

Patients who require ostomies because of cancer are frequently past middle age. Colorectal cancer usually occurs in men and women older than 40, predominantly in those over 60,[1] and advanced bladder cancer requiring a urinary diversion is more frequent in persons older than 50.[32] Questioning patients about how they have experienced events in their lives or coped with past stresses is important, because the answers may be predictive of how they will react to their current problems.

More time may need to be allotted to assess the support systems for older persons who require a colostomy or urinary diversion, since they are likely to have lost their spouse and contemporaries and to have a fixed income, posing greater financial concerns. Health professionals must be keenly sensitive to individual patients, however, and not assume that difficulties will arise. Some elderly persons who have survived many crises and losses are remarkable in their ability to handle stresses and unexpected events. For example, in studying cancer patients with ostomies, Watson[32] found that age of the patients did not affect their ability to handle the cancer/ostomy experience during the postoperative period. She did not, however, negate the possibility that age might be related to adjustment issues encountered later, after hospitalization.

Armed with knowledge of anticipated changes that occur with aging, health professionals can be alert to noting particular physical changes that affect older persons' ability to care for their ostomy. For example, joint changes accompanied by pain and diminished hand dexterity caused by arthritis or neurologic changes affecting coordination and sensation, encountered often in older persons, may interfere with their ability to handle ostomy appliances readily. If the assessment identifies such changes, the health professional can allow additional time for learning care of the ostomy, thus sparing the patient frustrations and discomfort. If the assessment identifies changes in visual or auditory acuity, integumentary changes, or a decreased tolerance for activity and concentration, health professionals can plan modified procedures and teaching sessions to promote positive interactions and to facilitate learning in a calm and comfortable atmosphere.

However, once again, in assessing elderly patients, health professionals must remember that each is unique; one cannot assume automatically that an older person has any or all of these problems. Although these are some of the common physical and psychosocial changes that occur in the elderly, individual differences predominate and require careful consideration on the part of health professionals. The active, highly motivated, and energetic older person is insulted, for example, if treated as physically impaired and requiring multiple accommodations or increased dependency. In contrast, however, someone who was inactive or a recluse when younger is likely to behave similarly as an older person, and unrealistic expectations for this person's social rehabilitation are inappropriate.

## Dependency

Patients who transfer to a cancer center from a community hospital or distant setting may desire so strongly to receive treatment and may see such a transfer so hopefully—or as a last resort—that they do not ask questions about techniques or procedures and are not assertive in seeking their rights. Some patients feel so dependent on their physicians and other caregivers that they avoid disturbing them or questioning them because they are fearful of jeopardizing their treatment. Health professionals must be alert to this potential problem.

The author vividly recalls accompanying a cancer patient to a large clinic that was overcrowded and had inadequate seating. In many instances, the patients and families stood for long periods without being acknowledged by the staff, and yet they neither complained nor investigated delays in appointments, but rather waited patiently. Their behavior seemed to document the desperation and vulnerability of the patient with cancer.

When health professionals are aware of this tendency in their patients, they can encourage more realistic and assertive behavior. Health professionals should see the patient as a partner in decision-making rather than as a compliant and dependent recipient of care.

## COPING WITH CANCER AND AN OSTOMY

Body image is the intrapersonal experience of feelings and attitudes toward one's body.[21] It relates to one's actual appearance and body function as well as to how one perceives oneself, how others perceive one, and what one perceives as an "ideal body."[8] Awareness of this multifocal definition of body image is important if the health professional is to understand the psychosocial adjustment needs of someone with cancer and an ostomy; patients with cancer and an ostomy have unique and appropriate ways of adapting to their altered body image and must do so at their own pace.

### Altered Body Function

Loss of a body function (i.e., the normal function of elimination) can be similar to the death or loss of a significant person. Because mourning for the loss of body functioning is expected, the health professional can anticipate anxiety, depression, anger, resentment, and some dependency during the postoperative period.[4,13] When decision-making produces anxiety in the patient, health professionals should take over and accept dependency temporarily. As patients recover, the goals of self-care and independent functioning need to be promoted; at this time the health care team should provide the psychological support and educational information essential for patients to attain these goals.[5]

Patients particularly need emotional support during the early postoperative period, when they first see and experience the functioning of the colostomy or urostomy. The reality of the alterations in body functioning comes to the forefront at this time, and some patients are overwhelmed by it. The health professional, by changing or emptying the ostomy appliance promptly and in a matter-of-fact and efficient manner, spares the patient a distressing early experience of leakage or odor of feces or urine and reassures him or her that ostomy care can be normal and routine. It is important, in this early period, that care providers not express any feelings of revulsion or disgust if the appliance does leak or if drainage from the ostomy is excessive. Patients watch the nurses and physicians closely for signs of revulsion at the sight of the stoma or at the care necessitated by it.[4] Health professionals who feel strongly that elimination is a disgusting event require assistance to show them how detrimental this attitude can be for a patient who is trying to adjust to altered functioning in elimination. Although patients may intellectually acknowledge a colostomy or urostomy as a therapeutic procedure, they may find fecal or urinary incontinence and the exposure of a normally private experience (i.e., bowel or bladder functioning) a repulsive situation.[4]

Because nurses are eager to facilitate self-care and independence after ostomy surgery, patients may interpret their actions as rejection, as not wanting to care for the ostomy. In this instance patients' *perceptions* of the event rather than the reality are most significant. Health professionals cannot make assumptions about patients' reactions to the cancer or the ostomy without verifying these perceptions with the patients. Patients need to be able to express negative feelings, doubts, fears, and anxieties to care providers, who must be willing, patient listeners and responders.[13]

## Helplessness

In contrast to patients who have ostomy surgery for reasons other than cancer—for instance, ulcerative colitis, where the surgery is curative for the disease—the patient with cancer of either the genitourinary or gastrointestinal tract may require radiation therapy, chemotherapy, or both after surgery. Thus, in addition to the surgical trauma, such patients have to cope with the helplessness associated with these additional therapies and the side effects often encountered with them. For example, the patient who has adjusted to some degree to a colostomy may now experience increased psychological distress as radiation therapy to the pelvic area induces diarrhea and compounds problems in colostomy management. Patients may become extremely discouraged and depressed, feeling that they have lost control over bowel function and will never be able to regain it. This is one of the situations that can instill a sense of hopelessness and worthlessness.

Mrs. X., an attractive 50-year-old woman, at home after colostomy surgery for cancer, asked for the services of an enterostomal therapist to teach her how to irrigate and control her colostomy. While assessing the patient, the ET nurse learned that she was receiving radiation therapy and was eating minimally "to reduce the amount of feces from the colostomy." The patient was immaculately groomed and robed, but said several times, "I feel like a *sewer*, draining all the time."

The ET nurse advised her that learning irrigation was inappropriate at this time, both because the bowel was extremely friable from the radiation and because she could easily be "set up for failure" due to difficulties in managing irrigation control during the diarrheal episodes that accompany radiation. The patient was able to accept a delay in the irrigation teaching. At the same time, the nurse provided counseling about nutrition and provided psychological support at intervals during the period of radiation therapy. Some improvement in bowel function occurred during this time, and the patient subsequently was taught colostomy irrigation as her method of management. She was so successful in this method that she soon returned to her job, feeling comfortable about herself and her ostomy.

Stoner[27] stresses the importance of preventing or palliating helplessness and suggests interventions such as setting realistic goals, sharing information about what can be expected, pointing out degrees of success achieved by an intervention, and helping patients accept a realistic explanation about why uncontrollable events have occurred. Health care providers must emphasize an individual's sense of personal control over experiences whenever possible and feasible and avoid interventions that promote dependency and lack of control.

## Coping Strategies

Mages and Mendelsohn[18] have identified three basic modes of coping with cancer: (1) developing techniques to minimize distress; (2) attempting to deal with the issues; and (3) turning to others. They recognize techniques to minimize distress as efforts to avoid, to forget, to control, and to detach oneself from destructive thoughts and feelings. They note that "the use of some variety of avoidance or denial is probably universal and is generally a useful and appropriate method of managing anxiety." To deal with the issues, the authors recommend seeking information about the illness, taking an active role in treatment decisions, and confronting and mastering cancer-related problems by active and direct means. Turning to others as a coping mechanism includes sharing concerns with others and seeking support and reassurance from family and friends. Mages and Mendelsohn go on to say that how a person copes depends on at least four major contexts: (1) the patient's age and stage of life; (2) personal characteristics (how the illness is interpreted, what it interrupts, and what the stakes are for the person); (3) the person's interpersonal situation; and (4) the realities of the illness.

Weisman[33] has described 15 coping strategies used by patients with cancer. Among these strategies are rational inquiry (seeking more information), mutuality (sharing concern and talking with others), affect reversal (laughing it off, making light of the situation), suppression (trying to forget, putting it out of the mind), displacement/redirection (doing other things for distraction), confrontation (taking firm action based on present understanding), and redefining/revising (accepting, but finding something favorable). Other coping strategies identified by Weisman include passive acceptance; impulsivity; consideration or negotiation of feasible alternatives; reducing tension with excessive drink,

drugs, or danger; disengagement; blaming someone or something; cooperative compliance; and moral masochism (blaming self, sacrifice, or atonement). Since adaptation and psychological status are not static, patients with cancer and an ostomy may fluctuate in their ability to cope with the ostomy and its ramifications. They may use any or all of these coping strategies at various times during the preoperative and postoperative periods and during rehabilitation.

Denial may be viewed as a phase of the coping process during which a person revises a painful portion of reality and substitutes a more agreeable form.[16] Denial often exists together with acceptance.[16] It can be healthy and helpful, and its appropriate use has a place in the rehabilitation of a person with a disability such as an ostomy.[5,6] Denial can be an effective coping mechanism as long as it does not interfere with obtaining adequate treatment or achieving rehabilitation.

The use of denial is illustrated by an attractive, energetic 40-year-old woman who had undergone four major operations for cancer in a year and a half. On several mornings going to work (as principal of a grade school) in a wheelchair necessitated by cancer metastasis, she announced, "Today, I do *not* have cancer. I do not want to talk about it or to have the word mentioned." Her statements reflected her need for relief from the all-consuming experience of cancer and for normalcy in her life, in spite of alopecia, nausea, pain, and other cancer-related disabilities. Her comments could have been misinterpreted, however, by someone who evaluated the statement out of the context of her total pattern of behavior, life-style, and personality. And yet this woman consistently showed courage and honesty in coping with her cancer and managing a remarkable quality of life until her death.

## Counseling

### An Ongoing Process

Krol[16] identifies two tendencies among nurses and other health professionals: one, to assess and diagnose a patient's psychological response as a static phenomenon, and the other, to believe that denying is not appropriate while acceptance is. "Capturing a moment of that process (i.e., the patient's coping or denying as an ongoing, dynamic process) does not adequately describe the process itself," she reminds us, and cautions health professionals not to make assumptions based on initial or infrequent contacts with cancer patients. As health providers get to know the patients better, they can confirm, verify, or contradict relationships and perceptions over time. Frequent relevant discussions are conducive to making appropriate evaluations of the patient's psychological status. However, Young-Brockhopp[35] cautions that some persons do not wish to discuss their feelings and points out that "paying attention to the characteristic defenses used by the individual may be much more important than arbitrarily encouraging emotional expression."

Watson[31,32] studied the effects of counseling sessions during the postoperative hospitalization of 31 persons after urostomy or colostomy surgery considered corrective for cancer. Watson's purpose was to explore the effects of ostomy surgery on feelings about the self and its perceived effects on future life events from the patient's frame of reference. Her counseling approach included empathic understanding, positive regard, genuineness, and concreteness. Counselors responded to feelings, content, and meaning of the patients' statements and also began to identify the steps needed for patients to achieve their goals. They emphasized problem-solving skills and a positive adaptive response to the ostomy.

Watson found that four sessions conducted by a rehabilitation counselor on a one-to-one basis had a positive effect in altering self-concept/self-esteem as compared to control-group patients who received customary postoperative care. She argued for assigning a higher priority to supportive postoperative counseling, noting that "counseling needs relative to the cancer/ostomy experience are likely to come to the forefront once physiologic status returns to a more normal state." This, she said, was a "propitious time to initiate a formal counseling intervention."[31]

### Goals

*Facilitate communication.* Facilitating communication and exploring reactions of the patient and family to the cancer diagnosis and ostomy surgery are essential for meeting psychosocial needs. Listening intently conveys interest in the patient and is supportive for the patient's self-concept and self-esteem at a time when the patient feels vulnerable. In contrast, body language that indicates the health care provider is in a hurry, such as standing at the door while asking patients about themselves, is certainly not conducive to supporting the patient's self-esteem. Sitting down and promoting eye contact are conducive to supporting the patient's self-esteem.

Health care providers should be advocates for cancer patients and intercede on their behalf. Reassuring a patient that emotional reactions such as anxiety, anger, and depression are common when one is adjusting to a cancer diagnosis and ostomy surgery, and that these reactions are not inappropriate or unacceptable, is also a supportive intervention.

*Reduce stress.* Reducing the stress associated with the double diagnosis of cancer and need for an ostomy is an essential task for health care providers. It may be embarrassing for these patients to talk freely about elimination, normally a private concern, so that providing a comfortable atmosphere for such a discussion is the first step. A major way of relieving stress is to help a patient learn to manage the ostomy effectively and gain a sense of control.

The counselor may teach techniques of imagery, meditation, and progressive relaxation, which have helped some cancer patients reduce stress, develop control, and relieve fears.[3,6,14] Cobb[2] supports the use of relaxation techniques to help patients with cancer cope with anxiety, pain, and the side effects of treatments. She proposes progressive muscle relaxation as an appropriate technique to teach patients, as long as they are assessed for readiness and there are no contraindications such as weakness and fatigue,[14] cardiac irregularities, severe depression, or psychosis.[3] Cobb's teaching plan for relaxation includes: (1) resting quietly in a comfortable position, seated or semireclining with all extremities supported; (2) gradually closing the eyes and then keeping them closed; and (3) after several minutes with the eyes closed, beginning the progressive tensing and relaxing of all muscles from the feet up the legs, trunk, arms, neck, mouth, and eyes. Rhythmic breathing is also used for 10 minutes.

Simonton et al.[25] have proposed using systematic relaxation and visualization as a means of altering the progression of cancer, not only by reducing stress, but also by helping the immune system to "fight against cancer cells." The Simonton psychotherapy method emphasizes the person's power of living or dying from cancer by changing his or her beliefs and improving self-image. The Simontons also suggest that patients may have unconsciously brought on their disease by their behavior and attitudes. Health professionals must be very careful in using this approach. For some patients, this method may add more guilt and an additional burden, especially if their condition worsens in spite of adopting this approach. Additional stress and guilt may only isolate patients further at a time of vulnerability, when psychological comfort and solace is what they need. The Simontons' method has been advocated by many health professionals, but no systematic studies have been done to document its results. The American Cancer Society has cited it as an "unproven method of treatment" because of no scientific basis for claims of efficacy.[30]

### Posthospitalization

Freidenbergs and coworkers[10] have identified three basic types of psychosocial interventions appropriate for cancer patients and their families at home, after hospitalization. These are: (1) education, to assist the patient and family to live effectively with the disease; (2) counseling, which allows and encourages ventilation of feelings and provides verbal reassurance and assistance in clarifying these feelings; and (3) environmental manipulation, which includes consulting with other health care personnel and making formal service referrals to appropriate agencies. For example, patients who base their self-esteem on their physical appearance or on fulfilling needs of others have more difficulty coping with cancer, the ostomy, and their temporary dependency and may need referrals for follow-up and more intensive psychological support. Patients who express extreme feelings of worthlessness over a prolonged time should be referred for psychiatric evaluation.[17]

It is important that members of the health care team recognize when the patient's psychosocial needs exceed their own capabilities for meeting them. For some patients and families, referrals for psychological or psychiatric consultation are appropriate. For others, early referral

to a home health agency, providing adequate information on the patient's physical and psychosocial status, is appropriate to help patients manage some aspects of care such as nutrition and pain and to provide emotional support. These issues, plus the need to "re-teach" ostomy care, are the problems most frequently encountered by counselors visiting cancer patients and families at home[19]

## SUPPORT SYSTEMS

### The Family

The entire family of the patient with cancer and an ostomy should be viewed as the unit of care. The family, defined broadly, includes not only the nuclear family members, but also significant others in the patient's network of social relationships. As family dynamics are altered by cancer in a member, roles are changed and usual communication patterns may be disrupted.

The family's needs and expectations should be assessed along with those of the patient. When the family is included in preoperative and postoperative care and counseling, the patient feels less isolated. If the family is not included, its members in turn may feel isolated and neglected, resulting in feelings of anger, guilt, grief, indifference, or over-solicitousness. Family members may perceive the patient to have higher degrees of symptom distress than patients themselves report.[20] Unless communication with family members is open, their anxiety may be transferred to the patient and negatively affect the patient's coping abilities.

Dyk and Sutherland[7] found that many of their patients concealed their ostomy from the spouse, citing fear of rejection, shame, modesty, and actual evidence of disgust as the reasons. The authors observed that depression, chronic anxiety, and a sense of social isolation resulted. The health care team must emphasize the spouse's participation in the patient's care and adjustment, especially since the majority of patients list the spouse as the most important significant other and the key to the patient's personal success or failure.[23]

Kobza[15] conducted a descriptive study of 20 spouses of patients with an ostomy and either colorectal or urinary bladder cancer. The majority listed the need for information as their primary need. Interestingly, nearly half of the spouses stated they had received no information about ostomy care; even when they had received some information, psychological or social implications had usually been ignored. The second most frequently identified need was that of support: emotional reactions in all age groups ranged from feelings of shock to a sense of relief or acceptance.

How the patient's illness will affect the roles and activities of other family members should be considered. Often family members are unable to express their needs or fears, so health professionals must reach out to the family, conveying interest, acceptance, assurance, and recognition of their importance. Concern for the welfare of family members can be conveyed by encouraging their appropriate participation in the patient's care. However, family members must meet their own needs for time away from the patient and for pleasant diversional routine activities without feeling guilty. They often need counseling to use their energies wisely and to avoid exhaustion from overcommitment to the patient's care. Otherwise, as their own needs are not met, they may become resentful or angry. When family relationships were good before the illness, they usually continue to be good and prove to be assets to the patient. When relationships within the family were poor before the illness, they usually deteriorate, offer little in the way of positive support, and may be frankly detrimental.[28,29] Referrals to family agencies accustomed to working constructively with family groups are appropriate for this latter group.

## The Health Care Team

Many health care providers share a negative view of cancer, associating it with mutilation, pain, suffering, and dependency.[17] They, too, must communicate openly with cancer patients to determine accurately the patients' feelings. Jennings and Muhlenkamp[11] studied 28 terminally ill patients hospitalized with cancer to determine their evaluation of three affective states: anxiety, hostility, and depression. They then compared these perceptions with the evaluations of 28 health professionals caring for these patients. They found that for each affective state, the caregiver rated the patient as feeling considerably worse than the patients themselves reported feeling. These investigators were concerned that caregivers' overestimations of cancer patients' psychological pain may be reflected in their interaction with the patients, by either showing overconcern or withholding honest communication rather than being open and pertinent. This behavior could induce feelings of isolation and loss of identity in the patient.

## Spiritual Resources

Spiritual care is another resource for meeting the psychosocial needs of cancer patients and for increasing feelings of security in many situations. To some extent, health care professionals can provide a supportive atmosphere in which the meaning of life, illness, and destiny can be discussed. Realistically, however, the important relationship between clergy and patients should be facilitated by providing the privacy and respect that are conducive to spiritual counseling. At the same time, well-meaning health care professionals should be cautious about promoting guilt or forcing religious contacts on persons who are not interested in formal religion.

## Financial Status

Financial issues become particularly important for patients with cancer when they must undergo repeated hospitalizations, costs of ostomy supplies increase, other treatments such as chemotherapy or radiation therapy become necessary, and when they must decrease their employment as a result of surgery or the effects of treatment. Often ostomy surgery is performed in elderly persons who may find it necessary to have their adult sons or daughters begin to take responsibility for their care and finances. Some families accept this situation positively, but others view it negatively as creating additional stresses and burdens on the families involved.

Some patients, after surgery, feel that they are unable to return to work or to the social relationships that employment involves, and therefore they evolve a pattern of social withdrawal—unnecessarily prolonged convalescence or early retirement.[1] On their part, some employers are reluctant to hire persons with a history of cancer—sometimes because, if they do, they may incur higher insurance premiums or reduced insurance coverage. For this reason cancer patients are reluctant to change jobs, even after curative surgery, so that their personal career growth suffers.[24] All of these issues have implications for the financial status of patients and their families.

## Self-Help Groups

In many communities, self-help groups are available for patients with cancer or with ostomies. Persons with ostomies vary in their need or desire for participation in such groups, but they should be informed of their availability, purposes, and programs. Meeting positive role models in such groups as the United Ostomy Association, "I Can Cope" programs, or "Make Today Count" may be particularly beneficial. Even if patients receive much support and information from health professionals, they may find a different and valuable support system in these mutual support groups. "I Can Cope" programs have been shown to alter patients' anxiety, knowledge about their disease, and their sense of meaning in life.[12] In fact, some people are more able to speak freely of their condition to casual acquaintances than to people close to them.[1] Patients with cancer and ostomies often feel isolated and find comfort in knowing that they are not alone in their situation. Problems are easier to confront and manage when patients can share concerns and frustrations and gain support from other people who have experienced the same diagnosis and surgery.

Ostomy visitors—persons who are coping successfully with an ostomy and volunteer to call on hospitalized patients—can be invaluable to a patient with a new ostomy. Their presence can assure the new patient that someone with an ostomy can lead a normal everyday life. Often patients ask questions of ostomy visitors that they will not ask of others.[1] However, just as someone with cancer and an ostomy has the right to know about ostomy associations, he or she also has the right to not feel pressured to join, attend meetings, or even to have an ostomy visitor. Some persons are very private about themselves. Characteristically they were not participants in group activities nor felt the need for them prior to surgery and do not plan to change now. Some persons, for example, have

close intimate relationships with a small cluster of significant persons and feel no need to seek additional support systems. Others, however, benefit immensely from these support groups, often establishing strong and meaningful long-term relationships.

## CONCLUSION

Adaptation to a colostomy or urostomy is deemed successful when patients are comfortable and secure in their new way of managing the elimination of feces, flatus, or urine and begin to broaden their social interactions and activities.[5] The presence of an ostomy should not impede physical or social activities unless the person has failed to learn to manage the ostomy properly, is in poor physical health, or has failed to adjust emotionally to the altered body image.

The person who is well adjusted after having an ostomy created as a result of cancer does not deny the presence of the ostomy, but also does not dwell on it or spend excessive time in its care.[4] Rehabilitated patients do not place undue restrictions on themselves because they have cancer or an ostomy, nor do they use the ostomy as an excuse for unsuccessful relationships.[5] Rather, the well-adjusted person with cancer and an ostomy resumes social relationships satisfactorily.

Most people, in spite of all the emotional trauma associated with cancer and the creation of an ostomy, learn to master their care. In fact, many report that their confrontation with cancer has led to reevaluation of their lives and values and to much deeper and richer life experiences.[16] Others report a greater appreciation of life, a more positive attitude toward living, and increased self-esteem.[9]

This author has been impressed by the motivation, resilience, and strengths of many patients of all ages with cancer-caused ostomies who have adapted to the crises in their lives with ingenuity, courage, and perseverance. In some instances patients have developed more satisfying relationships with significant others because they have united in a concerted effort to cope with the challenges imposed by cancer and an ostomy.

## REFERENCES

1. Broadwell DC, Jackson BS (Eds): Principles of Ostomy Care. St. Louis, C. V. Mosby, 1982
2. Cobb SC: Teaching relaxation techniques to cancer patients. Cancer Nurs 7:157–161, 1984
3. Donovan M: Relaxation with guided imagery: A useful technique. Cancer Nurs 3:27–32, 1980
4. Dudas S: Postoperative considerations, in Broadwell DC, Jackson BS (Eds): Principles of Ostomy Care. St. Louis, C. V. Mosby, 1982, pp 340–368
5. Dudas S: Rehabilitation concepts of nursing. J Enterostom Ther 11(1):6–15, 1984
6. Dunlop JC: Critical problems facing young adults with cancer. Oncol Nurs Forum 9(3):33–38, 1982
7. Dyk RB, Sutherland AM: Adaptation of the spouse and other family members to the colostomy patient. Cancer 9:123–138, 1956
8. Fisher SG: The psychosexual effects of cancer and cancer treatment. Oncol Nurs Forum 10(2):63–68, 1983
9. Frank-Stromberg M, Wright P: Ambulatory cancer patients' perceptions of the physical and psychosocial changes in their lives since the diagnosis of cancer. Cancer Nurs 7:117–130, 1984
10. Freidenbergs I, Gordon W, Hibarrd MR, Diller L: Assessment and treatment of psychosocial problems of the cancer patient: A case study. Cancer Nurs 3:111–119, 1980
11. Jennings BM, Muhlenkamp AF: Systematic misperception: Oncology patients' self-reported affective states and their care-givers' perceptions. Cancer Nurs 4:485–489, 1982
12. Johnson J: The effects of patient education course on persons with a chronic illness. Cancer Nurs 5:117–123, 1982
13. Joson RO, Glitierrez R: Problems of rehabilitation of Filipino stoma patients. J Enterostom Ther 10(5):161–165, 1983
14. Kaempfer S: Relaxation training reconsidered. Oncol Nurs Forum 9:16–18, 1982
15. Kobza L: Impact of ostomy upon the spouse. J Enterostom Ther 10(2):54–57, 1983
16. Krol MA: The patient with cancer, in Beyers M, Dudas S: The Clinical Practice of Medical-Surgical Nursing (ed 2). Boston, Little, Brown, 1984, pp 247–307
17. Krumm S: Psychosocial adaptation of the adult with cancer. Nurs Clin North Am 17:729–737, 1982
18. Mages NL, Mendelsohn GA: Effects of cancer on patients' lives: A personological approach, in Stone GC, Cohen F, Adler NE, et al (Eds): Health Psychology: A Handbook. San Francisco, Jossey Bass, 1979, pp 255–284
19. May DM, Oleske D, Justo-Ober PK, Heide E: The role of the areawide oncology nurse coordinator in the home care of cancer patients. Oncol Nurs Forum 9(4):39–43, 1982
20. McCorkle R, Young K: Development of a symptom-distress scale. Cancer Nurs 1:373–378, 1978
21. Norris CM: Body image, its relevance to professional nursing, in Carlson CE, Blackwell B (Eds): Behavioral Concepts and Nursing Intervention. Philadelphia, J. B. Lippincott, 1978
22. O'Neill M: Psychological aspects of cancer recovery. Cancer 36:271–273, 1975
23. Prudden J: Psychological problems following ileostomy and colostomy. Cancer 29:219–238, 1971
24. Roberts L: Cancer Today: Origins, Prevention, and Treatment. Washington, Institute of Medicine/National Academy Press, 1984
25. Simonton OC, Matthews-Simonton S, Creighton J: Getting Well Again. A Step-by-Step Guide to Overcoming Cancer for Patients and Their Families. Los Angeles, J. P. Tarcher, 1978
26. Sontag S: Illness as Metaphor. New York, Vintage Books, 1979
27. Stoner C: Learned helplessness: Analysis and applications. Oncol Nurs Forum 12(1):31–35, 1985
28. Sutherland AM: Classics in oncology. Psychological impact of cancer and its therapy. CA 31:159–170, 1981
29. Sutherland AM, Orback CE, Dyk RB, Bard M: The psychological impact of cancer and cancer surgery. Part 1. Adaptation to the dry colostomy: Preliminary report and summary of findings. Cancer 5:857–872, 1952
30. Unproven methods of cancer management: O. Carl Simonton. CA 32:58–61, 1982
31. Watson PG: The effects of short-term postoperative counseling on cancer ostomy patients. Cancer Nurs 6:21–29, 1983
32. Watson PG: Postoperative counseling for cancer/ostomy patients. J Enterostom Ther 10(3):84–91, 1983
33. Weisman AD: Coping with Cancer. New York, McGraw-Hill, 1979
34. Weisman A, Worden JW: Existential plight in cancer: Significance of the first 100 days. Int J Psychiatry Med 7:1–15, 1976–1977
35. Young-Brockhopp D: Cancer patients' perceptions of five psychosocial needs. Oncol Nurs Forum 9(4):31–35, 1982

Leslie R. Schover

# 7

# Sexual Rehabilitation of the Ostomy Patient

Cancer operations that create an ostomy are necessary for survival. When the goal of treatment is to eradicate cancer, the health care team expects the patient to return to all normal activities. Even if surgery is palliative in intent, we expect the ostomy to help the patient be more comfortable. However, most patients who are told they need an ostomy do not see how it can improve their life-style. Rather they view the stoma and appliance as a burden and a disfigurement, a permanent reminder of their illness.

In this chapter we describe techniques for helping men and women to integrate an ostomy into their self-concept and to continue feeling desirable and lovable. We also examine sexual dysfunctions that may accompany the surgery for pelvic cancer and suggest options for rehabilitation.

The literature on psychological and sexual adjustment after surgery to create an ostomy is sparse. Published studies have focused on small samples of patients, mixed in type of disease and site of ostomy.[12,15] Instead of relying on the literature, therefore, this chapter is based on our experience for the last three years in the Section of Sexual Rehabilitation at The University of Texas M. D. Anderson Hospital and Tumor Institute at Houston.

## THE PSYCHOSEXUAL IMPACT
## OF AN OSTOMY

Having an ostomy can affect a person's self-esteem and relationships through a variety of psychological mechanisms.

THE CANCER PATIENT WITH AN OSTOMY
ISBN 0-8089-1807-9

### Body Image

Of course the most striking aspect is the person's reaction to the loss of the bladder or the rectum, to the appearance of the stoma, to the appliance and its daily care, and to the surgical scars. At first the stoma and appliance feel foreign. Only gradually do they become a part of the person's self-concept. Sexuality cannot be separated from feeling attractive and desirable. Men and women with ostomies not only fear embarrassment in public from odors, bowel sounds, or a leaking appliance, but they must confront their anxieties about the mate's reaction to the ostomy at the most intimate moments.

In our society, the genitals are considered a taboo area. The fluids connected with sexuality, i.e., semen and vaginal lubrication, are often considered "dirty" along with urine and feces. Operations that alter bowel and bladder function may also have physiologic effects on sexual function. All of these circumstances can combine to make a man or woman feel that it is impossible to be sexually attractive or active when one has an ostomy. A statement heard commonly from surgeons and echoed by patients is, "After this operation, your sex life is over."

### Fear of Rejection

Men or women with ostomies often fear that their spouse will abandon them, or, if they are single, that nobody will ever want them as a sexual partner. Most spouses are actually quite supportive. Only a minority express great distress at looking at the surgical scars or at touching the stoma. Perhaps the goal of the surgery in curing cancer accounts for some of this acceptance. Spouses often say, "I'm just so glad to have him (or her) alive, that the bag doesn't bother me at all." In our experience, a strong negative reaction on the spouse's part often signals a history of marital conflict. Nevertheless, even in the most supportive relationship, most patients need several months before they feel secure about being accepted.

### Stress and Sexuality

To say that the diagnosis of cancer and the experience of pelvic surgery is stressful is to belabor the obvious. The anxiety about prognosis, physical pain of special examinations and postsurgical recovery, and fatigue from trying to cope with daily life combine to make sexuality a low priority. Little energy is available for expression of affection or enjoyment of leisure activities.

Sex becomes more salient, however, as recovery from surgery progresses. The wish to resume sexual activity parallels the desire to return to a normal life-style, to forget the cancer and feel whole again. For the man or woman with an ostomy, sexual desire often returns gradually along with the confidence that the appliance is relatively leakproof and is acceptable to the mate. Steps in this evolution include feeling comfortable being seen nude, sleeping in the same bed as the partner, and returning to a normal social schedule.

### Depression and Sexuality

Loss of desire for sex is one of the most common symptoms of a clinical depression, along with sleep disturbance, loss of appetite for food, depressed mood, feelings of guilt and worthlessness, irritability, and a wish to be alone. From a psychological standpoint, depression may be triggered by the loss of the many daily pleasurable activities in a person's normal routine or by the sense of helplessness and lack of control over the cancer.

Patients undergoing pelvic cancer surgery may experience depression not only as a psychological reaction to their disease but also as a side effect of medications, stress, anesthesia, or metabolic imbalance. When a man or woman does complain of a loss of interest in sex, it is important to look for other symptoms of an affective disorder.

### Marital Conflict and Sexuality

Sex cannot be separated from the marital relationship. If cancer treatment disrupts a marriage, sexuality is usually disrupted too. When surgery creates a medical problem in sexual function, a flexible couple can cope, but a couple already in conflict may fall apart. Some of the factors that help a couple deal with a change in life-style and sexual function include the ability to talk openly about feelings, good negotiating skills in making decisions about daily routines, a sense of humor, clear sexual communication, and comfort with a variety of types of sexual stimulation.

### THE PHYSIOLOGIC IMPACT OF SURGERY ON SEXUAL FUNCTION

### The Sexual Response Cycle

In order to understand why some cancer operations damage sexual function, one needs a basic knowledge of the sexual response cycle (Table 7-1) and the physiologic systems contributing to each phase (Fig. 7-1).

*Sexual desire* is the motivation to have sex. It can be measured only indirectly by a man's or woman's wish for sex, frustration when deprived, and actions in initiating sex or masturbating. Physiologically, the androgens influence sexual desire in both men and women. When androgen levels are abnormally low, sexual desire is usually low or absent. Surgical procedures that necessitate an ostomy generally do not include removing the testicles, a man's major source of androgen, but stress may temporarily reduce androgen levels.[25] Testosterone production should recover along with physical strength after surgery, however. In women, the ovaries are often removed as part of pelvic cancer surgery, but the adrenal androgens should be sufficient to maintain normal female sexual desire.

*Sexual arousal*, the next phase of the cycle, involves subjective excitement, genital pleasure,

**Table 7-1**
The Sexual Response Cycle

| Phase I Desire | Phase II Arousal | Phase III Orgasm |
|---|---|---|
| *Subjective Events* | *Subjective Events* | *Subjective Events* |
| Awareness of motivation to engage in sexual activity. | Awareness of pleasurable genital sensations and mental sexual excitement. | Sensation of orgasmic pleasure, preceded in men by the "point of no return" at the moment of emission. |
| *Physiologic Events* | *Physiologic Events* | *Physiologic Events* |
| Central nervous system activity, probably dependent on normal levels of circulatory androgens and prolactin and on brain dopamine levels. | Generalized physiologic arousal mediated by the autonomic nervous system (increase in heart rate, respiration, sweating). Vasocongestion of the genitals (erection in men, vaginal expansion and lubrication in women), mediated by a combination of parasympathetic and sympathetic nervous system activation. | In men, emission occurs, including contractions of the smooth muscle of the prostate, seminal vesicles, and vasa deferentia to transport mature spermatozoa and deposit semen in the posterior urethra. Bladder neck closes. Emission mediated by short adrenergic neurons of the sympathetic nervous system. In men and women, rhythmic contractions of the striated muscles in the genital area accompanied by the sensation of orgasm. Mediated by the sensory nervous system (pudendal nerve). |

and vascular engorgement of the genitals. In men, erection is the hallmark of arousal. In women, vaginal lubrication and expansion are perhaps the most salient features. Heart rate and respiration speed up and blood pressure increases in both men and women.

Arousal requires input from several physiologic systems: (1) the sensory nerves, especially the pudendal nerve that transmits sensation from the genital area; (2) the parasympathetic nerves that control blood flow to the genitals; (3) the short adrenergic neurons and perhaps peptidergic neurons of the sympathetic nervous system located within the penis and the vaginal walls; and (4) the pelvic vascular bed. Surgery for pelvic cancers in men is notorious for damaging the parasympathetic plexus around the prostate gland.[24,35] These surgical procedures do not damage the sensory nerves, however. Genital sensation remains normal. The role of pelvic surgery in reducing circulation to the penis or vaginal area, or indeed in affecting vaginal lubrication by any mechanism, is not clear.

The *orgasm* phase of the response cycle also has several components. The pleasurable

sensation of orgasm depends peripherally on input from the pudendal nerve, but also is a central nervous system phenomenon. In both men and women, orgasmic pleasure is usually accompanied by contractions of striated muscles in the genital area, controlled again by the pudendal nerve. In the male orgasm, these muscle contractions are the ejaculation mechanism that propels semen through the urethra. These two aspects of orgasm, pleasure and muscular contractions, are not damaged by surgical procedures that lead to the need for an ostomy.

In men, however, the emission component of orgasm may be disrupted. Emission is felt subjectively as the "point of no return" before ejaculation begins. Objectively, the prostate, seminal vesicles, and vasa deferentia are contracting while the bladder neck shuts tightly. The semen and sperm cells are mixed and deposited in the posterior urethra, ready for ejaculation.

Abdominoperineal resection often damages sympathetic nerves in the presacral area that control emission. Either the prostate and seminal vesicles are completely paralyzed or, in a

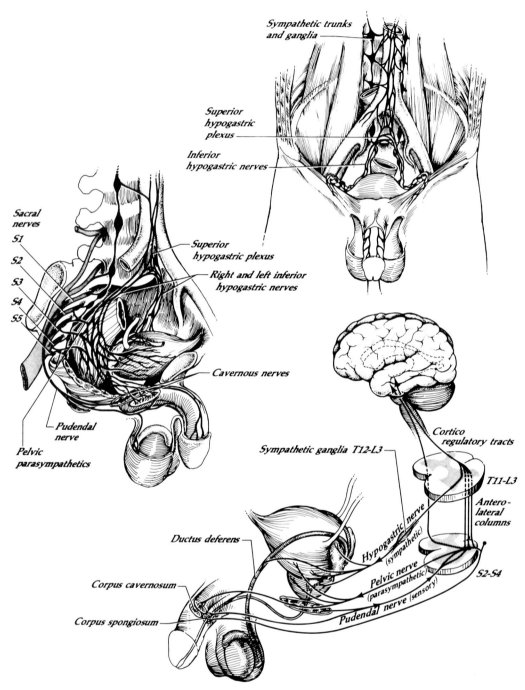

**Figure 7-1.** The neurologic control of sexual function.

less severe case, the bladder neck remains open and semen is ejaculated in a retrograde fashion into the bladder. In either situation, the result is a dry orgasm. Most men say the intensity of their pleasure remains the same or is just mildly reduced. No painful sensation occurs.

When men have a radical cystectomy or a total pelvic exenteration, the prostate and seminal vesicles are removed, again resulting in a dry orgasm. Many men still say their orgasm feels normal, but others report a lessening of the intensity of pleasure. A few men have told us that their orgasms become more prolonged and pleasurable after surgery.

In women, no clear equivalent of the emission phase exists. Our clinical experience in interviewing women before and after radical pelvic surgery suggests that as long as the clitoris and part of the vagina are intact, orgasms do not change in quality or frequency.[31]

## Sexual Function after Specific Surgical Procedures

It may be helpful to describe sexual function after each of the surgical procedures that commonly lead to creating an ostomy in a patient with cancer.

### Abdominoperineal Resection in Men

A man's sexual desire should remain intact after abdominoperineal resection because the testicles are not damaged. The lower colon and rectum are removed, necessitating a colostomy. A decrease in desire may be the result of psychological distress about the cancer diagnosis or about the colostomy itself. Genital sensation is normal after surgery, but the parasympathetic nerves that control blood flow to the penis are often damaged when the prostate is dissected off the rectum, creating erectile dysfunction. Several studies[3,7,36] suggest that the incidence of erection problems is not as high after this operation as it is after radical prostatectomy or cystectomy, however.

Men experience a high rate of dry orgasm after abdominoperineal resection. Reflecting the colon in the presacral area often damages the sympathetic nerves controlling emission. We do not know how often the dry orgasm represents a complete failure of emission and how often it is due to retrograde ejaculation. In fact, published studies really give no adequate estimate of rates of erectile dysfunction or of dry orgasm in this group of men.

### Radical Cystectomy in Men

After radical cystectomy sex hormone levels, and thus sexual desire, should be unaffected. Penile sensation and the ability to reach the sensation of orgasm also remain intact. The striated muscle contractions of ejaculation still occur,[6] but no semen is produced since the prostate, seminal vesicles, and proximal vasa deferentia are removed along with the bladder and prostatic urethra.

In our clinical experience, about half of the men report a full-intensity orgasm after cystectomy while half say their pleasure is reduced. Only rarely have we had a patient who could not reach orgasm at all, and then the cause is almost always inadequate type or duration of sexual stimulation. In other words, some men have reached orgasm always through vaginal intercourse, and are too embarrassed to try masturbation or to ask a partner to manually or orally caress the penis.

The incidence of erectile dysfunction after radical cystectomy has been reported to be about 85 percent.[32] Among our patients, at least a third of men have erection problems before cancer diagnosis (Schover LR, von Eschenbach AC, unpublished data), often, in this elderly group, because of such organic factors as antihypertensive medications, diabetes, alcoholism, or arteriosclerosis. If men have normal erectile function at the time of surgery, however, recovery rates for full erections in younger men, especially men under 50, may be higher than 15 percent. Most of our patients do have partial erections after cystectomy, but only a few can achieve sufficient rigidity for intercourse. Perhaps the use of surgical techniques described by Walsh et al.[35] to avoid damaging the nerves of the prostatic plexus will increase recovery rates. Only time will tell, however, if these new procedures are effective both in preserving erectile function and in eradicating the cancer.

When the bladder cancer is multifocal transitional cell carcinoma, or if the urethra is involved, a complete urethrectomy may be performed. No data are available on the impact of this operation on sexual function. We have not observed any clear effects of urethrectomy on recovery of erections or on the ability to reach orgasm. We have seen some men whose penis remains tender for up to a year after urethrectomy, however. This pain can delay implantation of a penile prosthesis. If a prosthesis is inserted, a semirigid one may not be as successful as an inflatable one; the semirigid prosthesis cannot compensate as completely as an inflatable for minor loss in penile circumference from removal of the corpus spongiosum. The glans penis is also more mobile than usual after a urethrectomy, so the surgeon may need to use special techniques to anchor the glans over a semirigid penile prosthesis.

### Total Pelvic Exenteration in Men

Total pelvic exenteration is such a rare operation for men that no studies of postoperative sexual function have been published. When it is performed, the operation's goal is usually to eradicate a large sarcoma of the prostate or a carcinoma of the colon adjacent to or invading the bladder or prostate. The margins of surgery include the bladder, prostate, prostatic urethra, seminal vesicles, proximal vasa deferentia, rectum, and lower colon. Two stomas are created, a urostomy and a colostomy. If possible, patients are taught to irrigate the colostomy, sometimes avoiding the need for two complete appliances.

Because of the extent of this surgery and also the type of tumors involved, men who undergo total pelvic exenteration in our institution are a relatively young group, often between 30 and 50 years old. Sexual function is thus a crucial issue in their rehabilitation. The recovery from surgery is often long and difficult. Many patients experience back and leg pain as well as genital tenderness.

Nevertheless, penile sensation and the ability to reach orgasm remain intact for most of our patients. Sexual desire also returns to normal levels. We have not seen anyone recover rigid erections after total pelvic exenteration, however. This is not surprising, since the crucial area between the prostate and rectum[24,35] has been completely excised. Like men after abdominoperineal resection and radical cystectomy, these patients are often good candidates for a penile prosthesis.

### Abdominoperineal Resection in Women

It is difficult to make generalizations about women's sexual function after abdominoperineal resection. The margins of surgery vary, but frequently include the uterus, fallopian tubes, and ovaries and occasionally the posterior vaginal wall, which is then repaired with a split-thickness skin graft. No systematic study is available of sexual satisfaction in women after abdominoperineal resection, but one team of surgeons has discussed surgical techniques to minimize the risk of dyspareunia.[11] They advise preserving the perineal body and using the levator ani muscle to fill the dead space behind the posterior vaginal wall. Their method may decrease damage to the autonomic innervation of the genitals and also provides cushioning for the vagina during intercourse.

Many women are postmenopausal at the time of abdominoperineal resection. Even if the ovaries of a premenopausal woman are removed, however, her adrenal androgens should be sufficient to preserve normal levels of sexual desire.[4] Because of the abrupt loss of estrogen, a woman may experience severe "hot flashes," which can disrupt her sleep and her sense of well-being. These symptoms may temporarily decrease her sexual desire. The other sexual problem caused by lack of estrogen is vaginal atrophy and dryness. All of these symptoms can be treated successfully with replacement hormones. Some physicians advocate a combination of estrogens and androgens to restore full sexual function.[8]

One question for future investigation is whether autonomic nerve damage during surgery results in reduced vaginal lubrication, even if hormone levels are adequate. A supplemental water-based lubricant can help to prevent dyspareunia when a woman's own vaginal lubrication is inadequate for comfort during intercourse.

The most common female sexual complaint after abdominoperineal resection seems to be dyspareunia. We do not know whether pain is related to the extent of surgery or to the operative techniques used. If intercourse is not painful, a woman should be able to reach orgasm just as easily as she could before surgery. Careful questioning of our patients before and after other pelvic operations, such as radical hysterectomy, has revealed that orgasm rarely changes in intensity or quality despite the loss of the uterus, fallopian tubes, ovaries, cervix, and even part of the vagina.

## Radical Cystectomy in Women

Radical cystectomy in women removes not only the bladder and entire urethra, but also the ovaries, fallopian tubes, uterus, cervix, and the anterior one-third to one-half of the vagina. At UT M. D. Anderson Hospital surgeons retubularize the vagina, using the tissue of the posterior wall. The usual technique is to join the cut edges of the posterior wall vertically, creating a narrowed vaginal barrel. Occasionally a surgeon dissects the upper half of the posterior wall away from the rectum and turns it downwards, creating a shallow vagina of more normal caliber.

We have interviewed nine women before and after radical cystectomy.[31] These patients were the only women, out of a pool of 39 treated during a two-year period, who had been sexually active before surgery. Women undergoing radical cystectomy are an elderly group. Many are widowed and have no sexual partner. Others have husbands in ill health who can no longer function sexually. Several studies of elderly couples have shown that the cessation of sexual activity usually depends on the husband's desire and ability to have erections.[14]

Of our nine active women, seven resumed sex after surgical recovery. All women who tried intercourse had dyspareunia at first, but over several months, six were able to reduce the pain to a mild level or overcome it completely. The pain was from vaginal dryness and tightness and responded to replacement estrogens, water-based vaginal lubricants, vaginal dilation, and psychological reassurance.

Women who resumed sex were all able to reach orgasm just as frequently as they had before surgery. The type and duration of sexual stimulation that allowed them to be orgasmic did not change. Even though the sensitive anterior wall of the vagina was missing, along with the underlying periurethral tissue, all six women who had intercourse were still coitally orgasmic. They did not notice any change in the subjective quality or intensity of their pleasure. Their reports cast doubt on the recent speculation that a special "G spot" on the anterior vaginal wall is crucial to a woman's orgasms during intercourse.[22]

Most of the women did notice vaginal dryness. It is unclear whether the decreased lubrication was caused by hormonal insufficiency, effects of the preoperative irradiation given to some women, or damage to pelvic autonomic nerves.

## Total Pelvic Exenteration in Women

Total pelvic exenteration in a woman is most commonly performed for cervical cancer that has recurred locally. Like total pelvic exenteration in men, it necessitates creation of a urostomy and a colostomy. Tissue removed includes the bladder, urethra, ovaries and tubes, uterus and cervix, the entire vagina, and the rectum and lower colon. At UT M. D. Anderson Hospital surgeons repair the resulting pelvic defect by using myocutaneous gracilis flaps to create a neovagina.[10] The vulva is usually left intact, unless disease in the vaginal introitus necessitates a vulvectomy as well.

As in men, the period of recovery and rehabilitation is usually long, even though many of the patients are younger than 50. Sexual desire is often reduced until a woman has integrated the ostomy appliances into her body image and has resumed as much as possible of her normal life-style.[2] The clitoris, if left intact, is usually just as sensitive to sexual stimulation as ever. Even women who have lost their clitoris have been reported to reach orgasm, however.[1]

The neovagina does not lubricate on its own. Most women need to douche daily to reduce vaginal odor. A water-based lubricant can make intercourse more comfortable.[10] Sensations during intercourse are different from before surgery. Some women report that caressing of the neovagina feels as if the inner thigh is being stroked. Nevertheless, a number of women do learn how to be coitally orgasmic again. Others depend on breast or clitoral stimulation to reach orgasm, a pattern that is within the normal range of female sexual function.[20] Few women say that dyspareunia is a major problem, once the neovagina has healed fully. Because the flaps include muscle in addition to skin, the vagina is cushioned and stays open without needing any dilation.[10]

## PSYCHOLOGICAL PREPARATION FOR SURGERY

The time to bring up the topic of sexuality is at the treatment disposition session, when the surgeon explains to the patient the rationale for radical surgery. The spouse should be present at this visit whenever possible. Some physicians believe in concealing as much as possible about the sexual impact of the proposed surgery. They fear that a patient who expects adverse effects is more likely to experience them. We disagree strongly with this point of view. An informed patient can cope with sexual dysfunction with less anxiety. The physician can draw an optimistic yet realistic picture for the couple by stressing the aspects of sexual function that will remain normal and explaining the sexual rehabilitation techniques available.

We deplore two common practices: The first is the failure to mention sexual function except as a term (i.e., impotence) in the informed-consent form. The second is telling a patient, "Mr. (or Ms.) Jones, after this operation sex will no longer be possible." We hope that this chapter will make clinicians aware of the multifaceted nature of sexual function and the potential for continued pleasure after surgery.

The physician rarely has the time to perform the kind of sexual and marital evaluation that best prepares a patient or couple for surgery. That task is ideally delegated to a trained sex therapist (i.e., a mental health professional with advanced skills in assessing and treating sexual dysfunctions). Most hospitals do not employ a sex therapist as part of their staff, or even on a consultant basis, but a social worker or a nurse with specialized oncology training can often learn enough about sexuality and cancer to be of great help to patients in the role of "sex expert."

## Initial Interviews

Soon after the treatment plan is set, the clinician who performs sexual evaluations should meet with the couple (or with the patient alone if there is no partner or the partner is unavailable). For some patients, the loss of physical attractiveness and changes in sexual function are the most dreaded aspects of surgery. Many others, however, are still preoccupied with the cancer diagnosis and prognosis, so that rehabilitation of any kind seems distant and of minor importance.

We advise beginning the evaluation interview with a general assessment of the couple's background and current emotional status. No matter what their sexual attitudes are, they are more comfortable discussing sexual material af-

ter a sense of rapport and trust has been built between the interviewer and patient.

We usually begin by reviewing what we have learned from the medical chart about each partner's age, occupation, number of children and grandchildren, and the way the cancer was diagnosed. Most men and women become involved quickly if asked how they felt about the discovery of the cancer, their confidence in the medical care received, and their current judgment about prognosis. Each partner's fears and hopes about the cancer surgery and later ostomy care can be assessed, including beliefs about the spouse's reactions to the stoma and appliance.

Some questions that can reveal strengths and weaknesses in the couple's relationship include: What kinds of crises has your family handled in the past, for example, an illness, death, loss of a job, child leaving home, etc.? What helped you deal with that situation? What got in the way? Do you have any worries about how the family will cope with this crisis?

The clinician can then focus on the couple's relationship. If the patient is single, the clinician seeks a history of past and present close relationships. Interviewing a couple together provides even more information, since the patterns of communication and conflict can be observed directly. Some particularly helpful questions are: How did the two of you meet? What attracted you to each other? What are the strengths that have kept your relationship going? How does each of you express caring and affection? Every couple gets annoyed with each other now and then. When the two of you are angry, how does each of you show it? Is there any particular issue on which you disagree?

At this point, sexuality can be introduced as a topic. Begin with the least sensitive sexual material. General questions are often best: Tell me a little about the place that sexuality has in your relationship. How has the cancer diagnosis affected your sex life so far? How often do the two of you have some sexual activity together?

In order to predict how a couple will cope with sexual dysfunction after surgery, the clinician needs a description of the quality of their current sex life. Is one partner always the initiator? After surgery, the patient may feel too insecure to make sexual advances, and the partner may also fear initiating because it might be perceived as too demanding on the recovering spouse. Flexibility in initiating sex could thus be a strength in the relationship.

Can each partner ask for the kinds of caresses he or she prefers? The physical changes caused by surgery and the inconvenience of the ostomy appliance may necessitate changes in a couple's sexual routine. For several weeks or months, intercourse may be impossible or positions for lovemaking may need to be altered. A couple needs to communicate, preferably in words but at least nonverbally, to avoid painful stimulation and to learn new ways of giving pleasure to each other. Adaptable couples use a greater variety of caresses. One good predictor of whether a couple resumes sexual activity is the partners' ability in the past to bring each other to orgasm through manual or oral stimulation. Couples who have only reached orgasm during intercourse are usually more reluctant to accommodate their sexual routine to the postsurgical situation.

The interviewer can learn even more about the couple by taking the time to interview each partner briefly alone.[26] The clinician may preface this part of the evaluation with the statement: "Some aspects of sexuality are easier to discuss when your partner is not present. I'd like to spend a few minutes with each of you alone to give you a chance to express your individual points of view as fully as possible." In each individual session, the clinician can give the partner a chance to reveal material that he or she would like to keep confidential. These interviews are a good time to assess emotion-laden topics such as masturbation, any current extramarital affairs, and strong reactions to the cancer or to the prospect of surgery.

## Questionnaires

If the interview suggests that either partner has current or past psychiatric problems, some psychological testing may be helpful in deciding what kind of support, such as psychotropic medication or psychotherapy, may be needed during the cancer treatment.

If a question of organic brain syndrome exists, neuropsychological testing should be performed. To investigate the possibility of psychosis or affective disorder, the Minnesota Multiphasic Personality Inventory (MMPI) has traditionally been the test of choice. Recently, however, two inventories designed especially to assess the emotional strengths and weaknesses of medical patients have become available. One is the Millon Behavioral Health Inventory (MBHI)[16] and the other is the Psychosocial Adjustment to Illness Scale (PAIS).[9] Although computerized test scoring and interpretation are now available for the MMPI and the MBHI, ethically and practically all of these tests should be interpreted by a licensed clinical psychologist trained in their use.

Several questionnaires are available strictly to assess sexual relationships. One that we find particularly helpful is the Sex History Form,[28] a multiple-choice inventory that asks about various aspects of sexual function and aids in making a multiaxial diagnosis of sexual dysfunction. Clinicians who work with sexuality should become familiar with the controversies about diagnosing sexual problems.[28] Another useful questionnaire is the Sexual Interaction Inventory,[23] which is filled out separately by each partner but then scored using both sets of answers to generate a profile for the couple. It measures how accurately each perceives the other's sexual desires and assesses each partner's pleasure and acceptance of self and mate in sexual terms.

## Preoperative Sexual Education

Just as the ET nurse prepares the couple for surgery by showing the partners how the stoma and appliance will work, the sex therapist can use pictures and models to illustrate how sexual function normally takes place and what effect the operation will have. We prefer three-dimensional lifelike models of the genitals, especially ones that show a cross-section of the pelvis. The explanation to the patient should include the names of each internal pelvic organ and each part of the external genitals. The clinician points out the function of each anatomic feature and the changes that occur during the normal sexual response cycle. For example, we explain the mechanism of erection or the way the vagina expands and lubricates. The clinician may need to refresh his or her own memory on these facts.[20,21]

As part of this education session, the therapist can highlight those sexual functions that are affected by the proposed surgery. It is crucial, however, to emphasize the facets of sexual pleasure that will remain normal after cancer treatment. If the patient is a man, the various types of penile prostheses available can be introduced.

Self-help books can supplement this session. The author's book, *Prime Time: Sexual Health for Men over Fifty*,[27] gives an explanation in simple terms of normal sexual function in men and women, the effects of aging on sexuality, and the medical and psychological treatments available for erection problems. The penile prosthesis is described in detail, with guidelines on how to make a decision about having one inserted. Other helpful books include Zilbergeld's *Male Sexuality*[37] and, for women, Barbach's *For Each Other*.[5]

Many patients believe some common myths about cancer and sexuality. They fear that cancer is contagious through sexual activity, or that sexual activity has caused their cancer. Some believe that if they resume sexual activity, the cancer will be more likely to return. The education session is a good time to mention these beliefs and make sure both partners have accurate information.

## THE IMMEDIATE POSTOPERATIVE PERIOD

An advantage of having someone who is versed in sexual rehabilitation as a member of the health care team is that patient and partner can be visited during the postoperative recovery period. Such inpatient visits are often brief, since the patient may not have much stamina. The counselor can address some important issues, however, including: initial reactions of each partner to the ostomy incision; compliance with medical care, such as getting up and walking, using pain medications appropriately, and engaging in pulmonary toilet; couple interactions, including difficulty in sharing emotions, trouble negotiating family decisions, irritability, excessive cheerfulness, and overprotectiveness by the healthy spouse; and preoccupation with anxiety about future desirability or sexual adequacy.

*Case example:* Mr. B., a 72-year-old farmer, had a radical cystectomy. His wife, aged 68, stayed with him all day during his three weeks in the hospital. She also slept at night on the folding cot in his private room. Mr. and Mrs. B. had been married for 49 years and called each other "Daddy" and "Mama."

Prior to surgery, the assessment revealed that the couple usually engaged in sexual activity once a week. Mr. B. had no erectile dysfunction or other sexual problem, but Mrs. B. had some discomfort with intercourse because of postmenopausal vaginal atrophy. Her gynecologist had prescribed estrogen cream, but Mrs. B. stopped using it because of her fear that it would cause cancer. She sometimes used moisturizing lotion as a lubricant and had had several recent episodes of vaginitis. The clinician suggested that in the future she switch to a water-based lubricant that did not contain artificial coloring or perfume. Mrs. B. never initiated sex and was often reluctant to make love when Mr. B. suggested it. She believed her husband had more sexual desire than was healthy for his age.

After surgery, Mrs. B. annoyed her husband by her constant inquiries about his comfort. As soon as he could have food, she pushed him to drink and eat. Nevertheless, Mr. B. encouraged his wife to learn how to change his ostomy appliance. He hinted to the enterostomal therapist that Mrs. B. would be in charge of his ostomy care at home, despite the health care team's efforts to encourage Mr. B.'s independence.

When Mrs. B. was at lunch one day, Mr. B. told the sex therapist that the cystectomy would end the couple's sex life. "I'm not a real man anymore," he sighed, "and Mama, well, she'll just be relieved. She thinks we're too old for all that now." The sex therapist tried to get Mr. and Mrs. B. to discuss their feelings about sexuality. Mrs. B. said that sex was no longer an issue, and Mr. B. agreed with his wife. The sex therapist suggested that sex might seem more important when the couple got home and Mr. B. began to get his strength back. She reminded the couple that they could talk to her when they returned to the hospital for follow-up visits.

## THE FIRST THREE MONTHS AT HOME

One of the most difficult periods for men and women undergoing pelvic cancer surgery is the first three months after discharge from the hospital. Both patient and spouse may feel depressed as they experience the full impact of the ostomy care routine and the need for continued cancer surveillance. Men and women who must undergo postoperative chemotherapy may be particularly vulnerable to depression. Patients often cope with surgery by setting a goal of enduring just a few weeks of discomfort. They expect that life will then return to normal and are not prepared for further stress.

We alert couples to the possibility of "homecoming depression." We suggest they notify us if sleep disturbance, prolonged loss of appetite for food, and depressed mood become problems. We also advise them to set small goals for themselves that can easily be attained. Examples might be to take a daily walk starting with one block and adding a small distance each time, or to call one friend a day to get back into social circulation. With each success experience, the patient regains a sense of competence. The spouse can participate in this process, especially by remarking on the progress made.

Some counseling needs to take place before the patient is discharged from the hospital. If possible, however, the clinician can stay in contact with a couple, either through scheduled therapy visits or by phone conversations during the first months at home.

If a man or woman has difficulty accepting the ostomy appliance and feeling physically attractive in spite of it, working on body image may be appropriate at this time. Most people make minimal or no changes in their style of dress to accommodate the ostomy appliance. Sometimes, however, resuming active sports such as swimming, skiing, health club activities, or jogging becomes a challenge. The patient may feel embarrassed to be seen in the locker room or in a bathing suit, or may fear an appliance leak during athletic activity. When a man or woman does engage in active exercise, however, a sense of truly returning to normal often results.

The psychotherapist can suggest that a patient look at himself or herself in a mirror,[17] at first fully dressed, and later in the nude. The mirror exercise can help people come to terms with the sadness about their physical scars and yet still be able to appreciate all the aspects of their bodies that remain intact.

Resuming sex is another issue to address, preferably around the time of hospital discharge. Most patients are physically able to have sex again about six weeks after going home. We usually suggest that sexual activity be resumed gradually, starting with kissing and cuddling, progressing to taking turns caressing each other's entire body without trying to sexually arouse each other, gradually adding in more genital caressing, and only when nudity and touching are comfortable, helping each other reach orgasm through noncoital stimulation and intercourse. These steps are based on the sensate focus techniques used in sex therapy.[19]

The basic sensate focus exercise requires the couple to set aside an hour of time just for sensual touching. One partner begins by taking the role of receiver. The receiver of touch lies prone while being caressed for approximately 15 minutes, then turns over onto his or her back for an equal period of touching. The receiver's only task is to be aware of the physical sensations evoked by being caressed. The other partner is the giver of touch. The giver's job is to try a variety of caresses, ranging from light stroking to a deeper massage, focusing on all areas of the receiver's body except the breasts and genitals. The giver should also notice the pleasant textures and appearance of the receiver's body. When the receiver has been caressed on both front and back, the partners switch roles.

As the couple learns to enjoy the sensual and intimate feelings of being close, more touching of the genitals can be included in the exercise. On the first few occasions, however, the clinician should instruct the couple to limit their caressing in order to avoid setting off performance anxiety and focusing too much on the goals of becoming sexually aroused or reaching orgasm. Although these exercises have been described in many self-help books, couples may find it difficult to switch from expecting sexual satisfaction to enjoying sensual contact in itself. Often a clinician experienced in sex therapy is needed as a consultant if the exercises are to have the desired effect. Detailed instructions on these touching exercises can be found in *Prime Time: Sexual Health for Men over Fifty* (pp. 187–193).[27]

When a man has had pelvic surgery, he usually does not achieve full erections, especially at this early stage of recovery. The couple needs to change their expectation that sexual activity should culminate in intercourse. Partners can practice helping each other to reach orgasm through noncoital manual or oral stimulation instead. Some couples may even wish to experiment with a vibrator as a sexual aid.[17] The less a man focuses on having hard erections, the less his anxiety will impair whatever erectile function remains to him.

If a couple resumes sexual caressing, but at six months postsurgery is still unable to have intercourse because of inadequate erections, they may want to consider a penile prosthesis. We believe that the functions of penile prostheses should be explained fully to every man before pelvic surgery is performed, but not until this time is he ready to consider it seriously. Counseling for the prosthesis will be discussed in the section of this chapter on long-term follow-up.

When the cancer patient is a woman, the couple should approach intercourse slowly and without pressure to attempt penetration until the woman feels relaxed and prepared. Most women fear that intercourse will be painful after pelvic surgery. Indeed, the incidence of dyspareunia is high after both abdominoperineal resection and radical cystectomy.[31] When a neovagina is constructed as part of a total pelvic exenteration, vaginal pain is less common but vaginal sensations feel foreign and abnormal at first. In addition, the inner thighs may still feel quite sore. When the couple is ready to resume intercourse, a clinician should repeat reassurances that intercourse will not damage the healed vagina, even though some areas may still feel tender.

We advise couples, however, to try the sensate focus exercises before attempting intercourse. We encourage the woman to ask actively for the kind of caressing she would enjoy, which is often a departure from her presurgery pattern of sexual communication. As the couple's touching focuses more on the genitals, we suggest the man lubricate his fingers with a water-based lubricant such as K-Y Jelly, Ortho Personal Lubricant, or Transi-lube. At first he gently caresses his partner's genitals around the labia and clitoris. When she is highly aroused and feels relaxed, he can slowly insert one finger into her vagina. If she feels no pain, she can guide him in moving his finger inside her vagina. If some genital soreness persists, the step of exploring vaginal sensations may take several weeks. The man should be able to caress his partner's vagina with two, and then three fingers before the couple tries penile penetration.

We also teach the woman to perform Kegel exercises,[17] so that she knows how to relax the pubococcygeal muscles around the vaginal entrance. Involuntary tension in these muscles can exacerbate dyspareunia.[13] The pubococcygeal muscles are those a woman squeezes to cut off her flow of urine. In teaching patients how to perform Kegel exercises, we ask the patient to insert one finger partially into her vagina. As she squeezes the muscles, she should be able to feel the vaginal entrance contract slightly. Once a patient knows how to contract the correct muscles, she can exercise them at any time, without needing to touch herself for feedback.

Several routines for Kegel exercises have been advocated, all of which help a woman to be aware of the contrast between tensing her muscles and relaxing them. One simple method of performing the Kegel exercise is to contract the muscle and then let it relax, repeating the process ten times. A woman can practice twice daily, making the exercises part of her routine. The success of Kegel exercises in actually strengthening the pubococcygeal muscle is controversial, but the exercises are certainly useful in giving a woman a sense of control over and awareness of her vaginal introitus.

When a woman is ready to attempt intercourse, we suggest she sit above her partner so that she can control how quickly and how deeply he penetrates her vagina. We remind her to use the Kegel movements to make sure her vaginal muscles are relaxed before she inserts her partner's penis, and also to spread a good deal of extra lubricant not only on her partner's penis but also inside her vaginal entrance. At first the man should not try any thrusting motions at all. The woman can move her hips gently if she feels comfortable. It may take several of these sessions before a couple is ready for full-scale intercourse. With guidance and encouragement from a counselor, however, both partners can remain patient, especially if they are comfortable using noncoital caressing to help each other reach orgasm.

Both men and women can benefit from some commonsense advice on minimizing interference of the ostomy appliance with sexual activity. Patients who have a urostomy should always empty the appliance before starting sex, to minimize the consequences of a leak. Some of our patients, especially women, purchase a "mini-pouch" (eight-ounce size) to wear during lovemaking. Those who have an appliance with separate faceplate and pouch can turn the pouch sideways. Men or women who wear an elastic support belt on their faceplate can tuck the empty pouch into the belt to keep it out of the way. Others may prefer to tape the pouch to the groin or hip to stop it from flapping during intercourse.

People who have colostomies deal with some different issues. If a man or woman can irrigate successfully, a stoma cap or safety pouch is much less distracting during sex than is a full-sized appliance. People with colostomies may also wish to have sexual activity at a time of day when their bowels are usually less active. They can also avoid foods that produce flatulence.

With any type of ostomy, men or women usually feel more attractive when wearing a pouch cover (Fig. 7-2). Some of our patients sew them in fabrics to match their lingerie, or use colorful knit material. We even have one man who had a t-shirt shop print, "I love my bladder," complete with heart, on his pouch cover. Some people still feel self-conscious about allowing the partner to see the appliance or the surgical scars. Women sometimes purchase "crotchless" panties or teddies that cover their appliance but leave the genital area free. A short nightgown can serve the same purpose. Some men feel more comfortable wearing an undershirt during sexual activity or tying a sash around the waist to hide the appliance.

Many couples find that the missionary, or male superior, position for intercourse is not as easy with an ostomy, unless the male partner supports himself on his hands rather than lying flat on top of the woman. Some couples find that a small cushion placed just above the faceplate minimizes friction on the appliance and reduces the chance of developing a leak during intercourse. Others change the position they use for lovemaking. They may prefer to have intercourse lying on their sides, with the woman sitting on top, or in any of the multitude of other coital positions that inventive couples discover.

*Case example:* Mrs. Y. had a diverting colostomy to treat bowel obstruction by inoperable tumor. An attractive woman of 54, she was undergoing chemotherapy for her metastatic disease. She and her husband had a warm relationship with good communication. They had been sexually active several times a week and wanted to continue to enjoy their sex life as much as possible.

Mrs. Y. worried that she would feel unattractive unless her appliance was covered. We discussed alternatives, but she found that both she and her husband were comfortable with her nudity, and that wearing a lace-trimmed pouch cover was enough to make her feel desirable in sexual situations. She and her husband had often varied the positions they used in the past for intercourse, and were quickly able to find one that caused no pain to Mrs. Y. and was not made awkward by the ostomy appliance. Mrs. Y. continued her chemotherapy as an outpatient and remained as social and busy as she could. Her physician assured

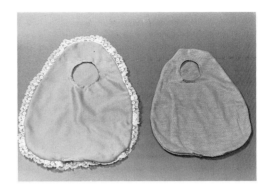

**Figure 7-2.** Pouch covers.

her that sexual activity was safe, even during her periods of immunosuppression.

## LONG-TERM FOLLOW-UP

Sexual rehabilitation is a long-term process. Even when a person appears to be completely back to a normal life-style, moments of anger or regret about the aftereffects of cancer are common. The ostomy is, of course, a constant reminder of mortality and of any handicaps the patient believes exist. Months, or even years, may pass before an appliance feels like an integral part of the body and before a man or woman can look in the mirror and focus on attractive features rather than surgical scars.

Both patients and clinicians should keep in mind, however, that the experience of cancer treatment can also have positive effects. Life usually seems more precious, and partners stop taking each other for granted. Cancer makes people reevaluate their priorities in life, often realizing that dreams they postpone may never become real. In terms of sexuality, the illness may make both patient and partner more aware of needs to express love and share closeness. The risk of asking for love, sexual or otherwise, may seem less frightening. Desires to experience more sexual variety and pleasure may also become salient.

Some special problems with sexuality call for intensive efforts at sexual rehabilitation. Unmarried men and women with ostomies may need considerable support and encouragement to begin dating again. Perhaps their partner at the time of surgery rejected them, or maybe the patient pushed a lover away rather than face the

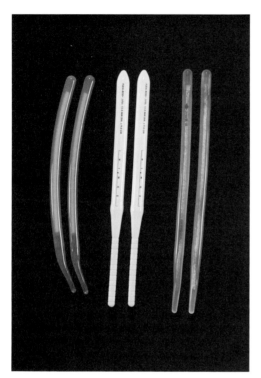

**Figure 7-3.** Types of semirigid penile prostheses: from the left, the Jonas malleable prosthesis, the Flexirod prosthesis, and the Small-Carrion prosthesis. (Reprinted with permission from A. C. von Eschenbach, L. R. Schover: Sexual rehabilitation of cancer patients, in A. E. Gunn (Ed): Cancer Rehabilitation, New York, Raven Press, 1984.[33])

vulnerability of asking for acceptance. The threat of a cancer recurrence makes it difficult to plan for the future and to make serious commitments. Young patients may be infertile because of surgery, radiation therapy, or chemotherapy.

To the public at large, a man or woman with an ostomy appears untouched by illness. Yet when the patient meets a potential mate, at some point the "secret" of cancer treatment and physical changes must be disclosed. This task is especially delicate because the surgery has changed the most intimate body functions, urination or defecation as well as sexuality. No rules exist on what to say or when to say it. Patients can benefit from a support group, however, and from role-playing with a therapist ways of approaching new partners and of discussing having cancer.

Another special problem is sexual dysfunction that has not resolved within a few months after surgery. Sex therapy techniques can be effective in treating such dysfunctions, but at this stage the therapist must be a trained mental health professional. Most sexual dysfunctions can be treated in 10 to 20 sessions of sex therapy[18,20] that focus directly on the sexual symptom. Conjoint therapy is the most effective format, since a couple's communication patterns and power struggles are usually part of the problem. Sexual problems can also be treated individually or in group therapy, however. The most essential component of sex therapy is assigning homework: exercises in touching, communicating, and demonstrating caring that gradually build new skills across the weeks of therapy.

After surgery for pelvic cancer, some men or women may need help in relearning how to reach orgasm, using unfamiliar types of sexual stimulation. Women may also have to overcome severe dyspareunia that does not decrease with simple advice on resuming intercourse gradually. Techniques that can help to reduce dyspareunia include relaxation training, the use of graduated vaginal dilators, and prescription of replacement estrogens when appropriate.[13] A gynecologist and a sex therapist should collaborate in treating such patients.

Low sexual desire is another common problem for both partners and patients in the months after surgery. Low desire may be a symptom of a clinical depression, but it also can indicate marital conflict or a chronic problem that began during childhood in a family with disturbed patterns of intimacy. Problems of sexual desire are often stubborn and complex, calling for careful assessment and treatment.[18,29]

Finally, as the penile prosthesis becomes ever more popular, many men are electing to have one implanted after pelvic cancer surgery. Types of semirigid prostheses currently available are illustrated in Figure 7-3. Figure 7-4 illustrates the schema of an inflatable prosthesis. Unfortunately, the simplicity of the surgery makes a prosthesis seem to be a deceptively easy solution. Technically, both the semirigid and the inflatable penile prosthesis have high rates of success. Apparently 80 to 90 percent of men are satisfied with the results.[34] Follow-up studies have not been adequate, however, to answer questions such as: Do men return to levels of sexual activity that resemble their function before surgery? How happy are wives about the prosthesis? Are they as easily orgasmic during intercourse as they were before the erection problem began? What is the impact of the prosthesis on marital happiness? What emotional factors predict a good versus a poor adjustment to the prosthesis?[30]

We strongly advocate including the partner in the counseling and evaluation leading to a decision about implanting a prosthesis. We also believe that many couples can benefit from brief sex therapy before and after surgery. Figure 7-5 summarizes our system of evaluation and treatment for erectile dysfunction in men whom we are considering for a penile prosthesis. The details of our methods are available to the interested reader in a previous publication.[30]

Even when no special sexual issue appears to be present, we recommend scheduling a routine follow-up visit to assess emotional and sexual adjustment at six months to a year postsurgery. Even with the best of presurgical preparation and postsurgical counseling, some problems persist, and often the patient does not spontaneously ask for help.

*Case example:* Mrs. H., age 66, and her 69-year-old husband had a very happy second marriage of five years' duration. Both had been widowed before they met in a retirement community. When Mrs. H. was scheduled for a radical cystectomy, the sex therapist met with both partners and discussed sexual function after surgery. She also visited with the couple during Mrs. H.'s hospital stay, and developed a warm relationship with them.

Mrs. H.'s recovery was uncomplicated. By the couple's three-month follow-up clinic visit the H.'s had resumed noncoital stimulation and each partner was orgasmic. The sex therapist encouraged the couple to try intercourse, giving suggestions on making penetration easier.

She did not see the H.'s again for six months. They lived several hundred miles from the hospital and were being followed on alternate visits by their physician at home. When they did return, the sex therapist was surprised to learn that, after two somewhat painful attempts at intercourse, the couple had given up on ever trying penetration again. Mrs. H. was afraid that intercourse could split open her reconstructed vagina. Mr. H. hated the idea of hurting his wife.

The sex therapist again explained the use of a water-based lubricant and suggested ways to make penetration gradual and relaxed. She made a date to contact the couple by phone in six weeks. At that time Mrs. H. happily announced that she was having regu-

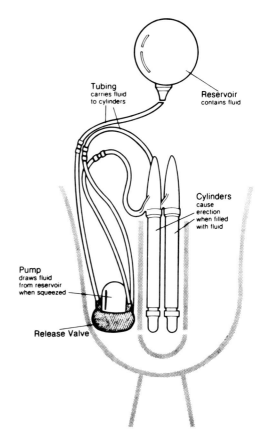

**Figure 7-4.** An inflatable penile prosthesis (American Medical Systems Model 700).

lar and pain-free intercourse with her husband. "Why didn't you tell me all those things before?" she asked.

## CONCLUSION

Pelvic surgery for cancer that entails creation of an ostomy can have a profound effect on both the emotional aspects of sexuality and the physiologic capacity for sexual function. Much of the psychological trauma can be prevented, however, by proper presurgical education and counseling. After surgery, sexual counseling can ameliorate the unavoidable emotional and medical side effects.

Sexual rehabilitation is not just a job for a specialist, but should be integrated into the treatment plan for each patient. The surgeon, the nurses, and the social workers should all participate in sexual rehabilitation by bringing

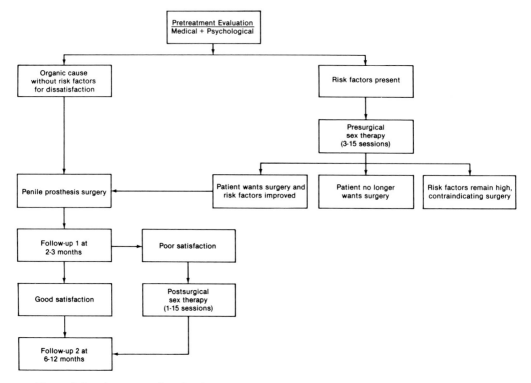

**Figure 7-5.** A system of evaluation and treatment for erectile dysfunction. (Reprinted with permission from J Sex Marital Ther 11:65, 1985.[30])

up the topic of sex, providing accurate information on sexual function, and making sure a patient has the skills and emotional resources to resume sexual activity in spite of the presence of an ostomy. Only when a man or woman feels attractive and able to be intimate with a mate can cancer rehabilitation be considered complete.

## REFERENCES

1. Andersen BL, Hacker NF: Psychosexual adjustment after vulvar surgery. Obstet Gynecol 62:457–462, 1983
2. Andersen BL, Hacker NF: Psychosexual adjustment following pelvic exenteration. Obstet Gynecol 61:331–338, 1983
3. Baklev I, Harling H: Sexual dysfunction following operation for carcinoma of the rectum. Dis Colon Rectum 26:785–788, 1983
4. Bancroft J: Hormones and human sexual behavior. J Sex Marital Ther 10:3–22, 1984
5. Barbach L: For Each Other. Garden City, NY, Anchor Press/Doubleday, 1982
6. Bergman B, Nilsson S, Peterson I: The effect on erection and orgasm of cystectomy, prostatectomy, and vesiculectomy for cancer of the bladder: A clinical and electromyographic study. Br J Urol 51:114–120, 1979
7. Danzi M, Ferulano GP, Abate S, Califano G: Male sexual function after abdominoperineal resection for rectal cancer. Dis Colon Rectum 26:665–668, 1983
8. Dennerstein L, Burrows GB: Hormone replacement therapy and sexuality in women. Clin Endocrinol Metab 11:661–679, 1982
9. Derogatis LR: The Psychosocial Adjustment to Illness Scale (PAIS): Introductory report. J Psychosom Res (in press)

10. Edwards CL, Loeffler M, Rutledge FN: Vaginal reconstruction, in von Eschenbach AC, Rodriguez DB (Eds): Sexual Rehabilitation of the Urologic Cancer Patient. Boston, G. K. Hall, 1981, pp 250–265

11. Entman SS, Coleman JL, Wilson G: Conservative coloproctectomy for the sexually active woman. Surg Gynecol Obstet 155:77–80, 1982

12. Follick MJ, Smith TW, Turk DC: Psychosocial adjustment following ostomy. Health Psychol 3:505–518, 1984

13. Fordney DS: Dyspareunia and vaginismus. Clin Obstet Gynecol 21:205–221, 1978

14. George LK, Weiler SJ: Sexuality in middle and late life: The effects of age, cohort, and gender. Arch Gen Psychiatry 38:919–923, 1981

15. Gloeckner MR: Partner reaction following ostomy surgery. J Sex Marital Ther 9:182–190, 1983

16. Green C: Psychological assessment in medical settings, in Millon T, Green C, Meagher R (Eds): Handbook of Clinical Health Psychology. New York, Plenum Press, 1982, pp 339–376

17. Heiman JR, LoPiccolo L, LoPiccolo J: Becoming Orgasmic: A Sexual Growth Program for Women. Englewood Cliffs, NJ, Prentice-Hall, 1976

18. Kaplan HS: Disorders of Sexual Desire. New York, Brunner/Mazel, 1979

19. Kaplan HS: The Illustrated Manual of Sex Therapy. New York, A & W Visual Library, 1975

20. Kaplan HS: The New Sex Therapy. New York, Brunner/Mazel, 1974

21. Kolodny RC, Masters WH, Johnson VE: Textbook of Sexual Medicine. Boston, Little, Brown, 1979

22. Ladas AK, Whipple B, Perry JD: The G Spot. New York, Holt, Rinehart & Winston, 1982

23. LoPiccolo J, Steger JC: The Sexual Interaction Inventory: A new instrument for assessment of sexual dysfunction, in LoPiccolo J, LoPiccolo L (Eds): Handbook of Sex Therapy. New York, Plenum Press, 1979, pp 113–122

24. Lue TF, Takamura T, Schmidt RA, Tanagho EA: Potential preservation of potency after radical prostatectomy. Urology 22:165–167, 1983

25. Schiavi RC, Fisher C, White D, et al: Pituitary-gonadal function during sleep in men with erectile impotence and normal controls. Psychosom Med 46:239–254, 1984

26. Schover LR: Enhancing sexual intimacy, in Keller PA, Ritt LR (Eds): Innovations in Clinical Practice: A Source Book, vol 1. Sarasota, FL, Professional Resource Exchange, 1982, pp 53–66

27. Schover LR: Prime Time: Sexual Health for Men Over Fifty. New York, Holt, Rinehart & Winston, 1984

28. Schover LR, Friedman J, Heiman JR, et al: Multiaxial problem-oriented system for sexual dysfunctions: An alternative to DSM-III. Arch Gen Psychiatry 39:614–619, 1982

29. Schover LR, LoPiccolo J: Treatment effectiveness for dysfunctions of sexual desire. J Sex Marital Ther 8:179–197, 1982

30. Schover LR, von Eschenbach AC: Sex therapy and the penile prosthesis: A synthesis. J Sex Marital Ther 11:57–66, 1985

31. Schover LR, von Eschenbach AC: Sexual function and female radical cystectomy: A case series. J Urol 134:465–468, 1985

32. von Eschenbach AC, Pamphilis TM, Kean TJ: Goals and potential for sexual rehabilitation, in von Eschenbach AC, Rodriguez DB (Eds): Sexual Rehabilitation of the Urologic Cancer Patient. Boston, G. K. Hall, 1981, pp 216–227

33. von Eschenbach AC, Schover LR: Sexual rehabilitation of cancer patients, in Gunn AE (Ed): Cancer Rehabilitation. New York, Raven Press, 1984, pp 155–173

34. Wagner G, Green R: Impotence: Physiological, Psychological, Surgical Diagnosis and Treatment. New York, Plenum Press, 1981

35. Walsh PC, Lepor L, Eggleston J: Radical prostatectomy with preservation of sexual function: Anatomical pathological considerations. Prostate 4:473–485, 1983

36. Yeager ES, Van Heerden JA: Sexual dysfunction following proctocolectomy and abdominoperineal resection. Ann Surg 191:169–170, 1980

37. Zilbergeld B: Male Sexuality. Boston, Little, Brown, 1978

Douglas E. Johnson, Christopher J. Logothetis,
Gunar K. Zagars, Dorothy B. Smith

# 8

# Special Problems Posed by Cancer Treatments

Special problems can and do arise in caring for patients whose ostomies are necessitated by malignancy. In previous chapters we have focused attention on the care of patients whose ostomies either were created as a part of a planned therapeutic attack to eradicate the cancer, were required to manage complications arising from treatments, or were constructed to palliate patients in whom the malignant disease had progressed to the point that it was causing severe symptoms or posing life-threatening problems. In this chapter we examine the problems that ostomies pose to those who deliver cancer treatments and the problems that these treatments may create in ostomy care.

Effective management of most malignancies today requires a multimodal approach that incorporates surgery, radiation therapy, and chemotherapy into an integrated plan. Obviously, the impact of these different therapies on patients with ostomies depends, in a large measure, upon the temporal sequence of their use relative to the ostomy construction. Problems that preostomy cancer treatments pose to the construction and maintenance of symptom-free ostomies have been discussed in Chapters 2 and 3. In this chapter, therefore, we limit our discussions to the effects of postoperative cancer treatments on ostomy care and the problems that ostomies pose for the delivery of these treatments. It is important that all members of the health team caring for these patients be cognizant of the multiple interrelationships between cancer therapy and stomal care.

## CHEMOTHERAPY

Cancer chemotherapy, by nature of its effects on cell division, injures both normal and neoplastic tissue. Table 8-1 classifies the more commonly employed anticancer drugs by their method of action. All of these drugs have side effects, some of which produce significant morbidity; they may be as life-threatening to the patient as the disease process itself. Consequently, those caring for patients who receive these drugs must exert maximal effort to prevent or reduce the severity of the side effects. This can be accomplished only when all members of the health care team are knowledgeable about the drugs and their potential effects.

In our discussion, let us examine the complex interrelationships of ostomies and cancer treatments from two perspectives: problems the ostomy poses to the oncologist who plans and delivers the chemotherapy and problems the drugs cause for the nurse and patient who must care for the ostomy.

### Problems the Ostomy Poses to the Medical Oncologist

The major problem that an ostomy poses to the medical oncologist is the increased risk of infection during periods of myelosuppression.

**Table 8-1**
Classes of Cytotoxic Chemotherapy

| I. Alkylating agents | II. Antimetabolites |
|---|---|
| A. Classical | A. Folate antagonist |
| Cyclophosphamide | Methotrexate |
| Nitrogen mustard | Dicloromethotrexate |
| Chlorambucil | B. Purine antagonist |
| B. Nitrosoureas | Mercaptopurine (6-MP) |
| Carmustine (BCNU) | Thioguanine (6-TG) |
| Semustine (methyl CCNU) | C. Pyrimidine antagonist |
| Lomustine (CCNU) | 5-Azacitidine |
| C. Antitumor antibiotics | Cytarabine (ARAC) |
| Adriamycin | 5-Fluorouracil (5-FU) |
| Daunorubicin | III. Plant alkaloids |
| Mitomycin C | Vinblastine |
| Bleomycin | Vincristine |
| D. Miscellaneous alkylating line | Vindesine |
| Cisplatin | Etoposide (VP-16-213) |
| Dacarbazine (DTIC) | Teniroside (VM-26) |

Infections occurring during leukopenic periods may arise from organisms already a part of the patient's altered bacterial flora or from external sources. Risks of infections from external sources can be reduced by appropriate prophylaxis, by having patients avoid people known to be exposed or infected with contagious illnesses, and by curtailing patients' activity in crowded areas such as movie theaters, shopping centers, and sports stadiums. Unfortunately, the infectious complications arising from the patient's own internal flora are far more difficult to avoid. However, if the oncologist takes appropriate measures to prevent infection and to monitor the patient's status, he can administer the same chemotherapeutic agents in the same dosages to patients with ostomies as to patients without.

Our treatment of a patient with an ostomy is based on the knowledge that the stomal mucosa is no different from the mucosa of the remaining gastrointestinal tract; all mucosal barriers, regardless of anatomic location, are subject to the same toxic influences of chemotherapy. However, patients with stomas are at increased risks for bacteria to gain entrance into the blood stream from injury to the stomal mucosa or from a breakdown at the stomal-skin boundary.

Before instituting chemotherapy, we routinely obtain cultures from the mucosal surface of the stoma and from any surrounding areas that appear inflamed, as well as from urine specimens. If the patient has an ileal conduit, a catheterized urine specimen is obtained from the conduit for culture and sensitivity (Fig. 8-1). These surveillance cultures are an absolute requirement for the safe delivery of cytotoxic agents and need to be repeated frequently throughout the patient's course of illness and of chemotherapy.

Before a patient begins chemotherapy, the peristomal skin area should be carefully inspected for signs of inflammation. If a *Monilia* infection is present, it should be treated with Mycostatin powder; if stool or urine has undermined the seal of the appliance and has caused inflammation, the faceplate should be altered to provide a more secure seal. The value of excellent nursing care is best measured here. Constant vigilance, accompanied by necessary changes in appliance configuration as the body habitus of the patient changes during the course of the illness, reduces the incidence of inflammation and the likelihood of systemic infection (Fig. 8-2).

Fungal infections are a particularly serious threat to myelosuppressed patients. Consequently, it has been our practice to treat vigorously patients whose cultures are positive for fungus (*Candida albicans*) with systemic antifungal agents such as amphotericin B before initiating chemotherapy. In the absence of inflammation, however, we do not routinely treat

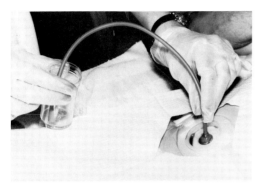

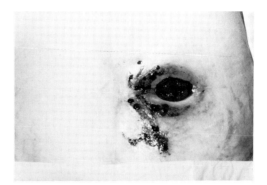

**Figure 8-1.** Sterile catheterization of an ileal conduit to obtain a urine specimen for culture and sensitivity studies.

**Figure 8-2.** The stoma of a patient who has a descending loop colostomy and is receiving 5-fluorouracil for colon cancer. When the stoma became slightly recessed at the edges, feces undermined the seal of the appliance and irritated the skin. The dermatitis is weepy and bleeding, partially due to the patient's low platelet count. A skin barrier and a slightly convex appliance corrected the problem.

bacterial growth in enterostomas. If virulent bacterial organisms such as *Pseudomonas aeruginosa, Klebsiella* spp., or enterococcus are identified during chemotherapy, we then institute antibacterial therapy.

One of the major benefits derived from surveillance cultures is that they provide the physician with the necessary information to begin broad-spectrum antibiotic therapy promptly when fever develops during periods of myelosuppression. The choice of antibiotics should be tailored to combat the organisms present in the surveillance cultures. Antibiotics are given intravenously and at full dose.

Our experience using aggressive myelosuppressive chemotherapy in patients with advanced bladder carcinoma who had previously undergone ileal conduit urinary diversion attests to the fact that cytotoxic drugs can be given in full strength to patients with ostomies.[11] The patients reported in this study were treated identically to patients who had not undergone urinary diversion, employing surveillance cultures and the guidelines discussed above. No fatal complication resulted from the treatment, and infectious complications, when present, were readily managed.

## Effects of Chemotherapy on Ostomy Care

The side effects of many cytotoxic chemotherapy agents directly affect ostomy care.[4] These effects may be generalized or very specific, requiring specific solutions.

### General Effects

Chemotherapy frequently potentiates an already present generalized asthenia, which makes it very difficult for patients to care for their stomas. In addition, a number of drugs (cisplatin, vinblastine, vincristine) can produce a peripheral neuropathy that reduces fine hand movements, further reducing patients' abilities to care for their stomas. Consequently, it is very important that the health care team constantly evaluate the methods of care patients are using and modify them when appropriate.

For example, if a patient has been irrigating a colostomy independently and now requires assistance, he or she should stop irrigating and manage the colostomy with a drainable pouch. This can be emptied as needed and changed once or twice a week. If a patient with an ileostomy or urinary diversion has been wearing a two-piece reusable appliance, a one-piece disposable unit (see Chapter 2) may be more easily managed at this time. These simpler methods of care may allow the patient to remain independent. If a patient is not able to provide meticulous care for the stoma, however, a companion should be taught how to care for the ostomy and the appliance.

## Specific Effects

Each chemotherapy agent causes its own specific side effects. Some of those that affect ostomy care are summarized in Table 8-2.

*Stomatitis.* Although many of the drugs cause stomatitis, and ulcers develop frequently in patients' mouths and other areas of the gastrointestinal tract, ulcers do not usually develop on the stoma itself during chemotherapy. However, the stoma may become very friable (Fig. 8-3) and require extremely gentle care. Stoma dilation (if used) and colostomy irrigations should be stopped until the stomatitis has cleared. Solvents or irritating substances should be kept away from the stoma. Each time the appliance is changed, the stoma should be examined closely for mucocutaneous separation or ulceration (Fig. 8-4). There is no specific local treatment for the mucosal ulcers; they heal as the systemic stomatitis resolves.

*Leukopenia.* Because many chemotherapy agents cause a decrease in white cells, patients must be especially careful to avoid infection. If a patient is wearing reusable ostomy equipment, it should be evaluated for cleanliness. Poor stomal hygiene and dirty equipment are never appropriate, but cleanliness is critical during chemotherapy. The cost of replacing worn ostomy appliances with a new set is nominal compared to 10 days of hospitalization, antibiotics, and the threat of septicemia and death. Disposable pouches may be the best to wear temporarily while a patient is myelosuppressed.

The oncologist may order a urine culture while the patient with a urinary diversion is receiving chemotherapy, particularly if the patient has an elevated temperature. If so, the culture must be obtained by sterile catheterization of the stoma, since a urine specimen taken from the appliance would be grossly contaminated and would not accurately represent the clinical situation. Occasionally a patient with an ostomy receiving high doses of chemotherapy may be placed in a protective environment to survive severe leukopenia. In this situation, the patient must use sterile ostomy appliances. Several disposable pouches, skin barriers, and accessories are available in sterile packaging from the manufacturers (Table 8-3).

*Thrombocytopenia.* Many chemotherapy drugs also reduce patients' platelet levels. Because the bowel mucosa is very vascular, the stoma may bleed easily while the patient has thrombocytopenia. Patients should be taught to examine the stoma, to clean the area very carefully, and to report any frank bleeding. Gentle pressure, cold compresses, or silver nitrate sticks may be used to control local bleeding. Suturing may be necessary and, in instances of severe bleeding, hospitalization and transfusions may be required. Petechiae may also develop under the adhesive area. The appliance should always be removed very gently to avoid trauma while a patient is receiving chemotherapy.

*Diarrhea.* Diarrhea can be critical in patients with an ileostomy. Because these patients have a delicate fluid balance, they can quickly become dehydrated and require hospitalization and intravenous fluid replacement. Patients who are receiving chemotherapy need to keep a careful record of intestinal output. They should be taught to monitor their output, if they are at home, and to notify the physician if early signs of dehydration appear. The problem is compounded if patients are nauseated, vomiting, or lose their appetite.

When patients who irrigate a colostomy for regulation experience diarrhea, they should stop irrigating and wear a drainable pouch until the diarrhea subsides. They should try eating foods that slow bowel transit time, such as applesauce, bananas, rice, tapioca, and creamy peanut butter. If the diarrhea is severe, medications such as Lomotil, tincture of opium, or paregoric may be required.

*Constipation.* Although constipation is not as frequent as diarrhea, some drugs can cause it. Symptoms can range from mild to severe; occasionally acute gastrointestinal distress and abdominal distention occur. A patient who is taking any of the agents known to cause these effects should be taught to be alert for constipation. If the patient is simultaneously taking pain-control medications, the problem of constipation is compounded. All of a patient's medications should be assessed together with the aim of preventing severe constipation. Stool softeners, mild laxatives, or retention enemas (see Chapter 3) may be necessary to prevent or relieve the problem. Once a patient has devel-

**Table 8-2**
Potential Problems for Ostomy Patients Receiving Chemotherapy*

| Problem | Drugs | Treatment |
|---|---|---|
| Myelosuppression | Adriamycin Cyclophosphamide 5-Fluorouracil Methotrexate Mitomycin C Cisplatin | *Leukopenia:* Use meticulous hygiene, clean ostomy equipment. Observe for skin breaks, ulceration, and signs of skin infections. Process surveillance cultures. *Thrombocytopenia;* Remove pouch gently to avoid trauma to stoma and skin. Observe for petechiae and mucosal bleeding. Avoid solvents or detergents. Avoid rubbing or friction when cleaning area. |
| Stomatitis | Adriamycin Bleomycin Cyclophosphamide 5-Fluorouracil Methotrexate Mitomycin C Vinblastine Cytosine arabinoside Actinomycin D | Cleanse stoma gently; avoid solvents and detergents; pat area dry. Discontinue irrigations and dilatations. No specific treatment: ulceration heals as systemic stomatitis resolves. |
| Diarrhea | Adriamycin 5-Fluorouracil Methotrexate | *Colostomy:* Discontinue irrigations. Fit with drainable odor-proof pouch. Recommend foods to slow bowel transit time (tea, bananas, cheese, applesauce). If severe, administer drugs to slow transit time (Lomotil, Emotrin, paregoric). *Ileostomy:* Watch for signs and symptoms of sodium, potassium, and water depletion; increase fluid intake (may need to be intravenous); record output. Check appliance seal. May need drugs to slow bowel transit time. |
| Constipation, ileus | Vincristine Vinblastine | Increase liquids, roughage in diet; may need stool softeners, laxatives, or retention enemas. If ileus occurs, administer no therapy orally; apply nasogastric suction and intravenous fluid replacement until ileus resolves. |
| Renal insufficiency | Cisplatin Cyclophosphamide Methotrexate | Fit urinary appliance carefully. Monitor output during overhydration and diuresis. Because methotrexate is less soluble in acid urine and can precipitate in the kidneys, discontinue urine acidifiers (vitamin C tablets, cranberry juice) during methotrexate therapy. |
| Neurotoxicity | Vincristine Vinblastine Cytosine arabinoside Cisplatin | Evaluate patient for problems of manual dexterity that interfere with ostomy care; simplify methods of care or teach a companion care of the ostomy. |
| Nausea and vomiting | Adriamycin Cyclophosphamide 5-Fluorouracil Cisplatin | Observe for signs of dehydration and electrolyte depletion; administer antiemetics; replace fluids intravenously; record fluid intake and output accurately. Offer small, frequent meals. |

* Adapted from C. Click, Cancer Bull 33:25, 1981.[4]

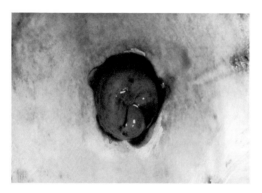

**Figure 8-3.** The ileal conduit stoma of a patient receiving combined cisplatin, Adriamycin, and cyclophosphamide. The mucosa is very pale as a result of the patient's anemia and the surface bleeds easily; it should be cared for gently.

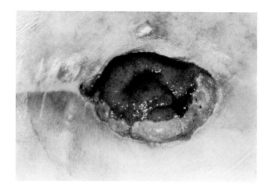

**Figure 8-4.** A patient receiving chemotherapy for leukemia had a loop colostomy constructed for bowel obstruction. Mucocutaneous ulcers and a whitish membranous layer developed during each course of chemotherapy. However, following each treatment the membrane sloughed and the ulcerated areas healed.

oped a paralytic ileus, he requires intravenous fluid replacement and restricted oral intake until bowel activity returns.

*Skin Problems.* Although any of the antineoplastic agents is capable of causing a skin rash or urticaria as a hypersensitivity reaction, some chemotherapy drugs may cause either a generalized or localized skin irritation unrelated to drug sensitivity, the appliance, or infection (Fig. 8-5). This reaction has been seen in pa-

tients receiving actinomycin D, Adriamycin, bleomycin, 5-fluorouracil, cyclophosphamide, and methotrexate.[1]

Determining the specific cause of any mucocutaneous reaction may be difficult, because cancer patients usually receive a combination of chemotherapeutic agents plus several other medications, including antibiotics, analgesics, and antiemetics. Immunosuppressed pa-

**Table 8-3**
Sterile Ostomy Appliances

| Manufacturer | Brand Name | Appliance | Cutting Range |
|---|---|---|---|
| United | Isotrol | Sterile wound pouch | 3 inches |
| Conva Tec | Duo Derm | Hydroactive dressing | 4×4 or 8×8 inch wafer |
| | Stomahesive | Wafer | 4×4 inch |
| | Sur-fit | Urostomy OR* set, accordion flange | 4 inches |
| | Sur-fit | Colostomy/ileostomy OR set, accordion flange | 4 inches |
| | Sur-fit | OR set 1 for urinary stomas, fistulas, or wounds | 2¼ inches |
| | Sur-fit | OR set 2 for ileostomies, colostomies, fistulas, and wounds | 2¼ inches |
| | Sur-fit | Loop ostomy system | 4 inches |
| Hollister | | Sterile postoperative pouch | 3 inches |
| | | Wound drainage collector, small and large | 3 inches |

* OR = operating room.

tients are especially vulnerable to a variety of reactive phenomena in the skin. These reactions may appear as an erythematous or as an acne-like rash. There is no real treatment for this irritation except gentle skin care and a skin barrier. The irritation disappears when the drug is discontinued. During chemotherapy, skin care should be very thorough, yet gentle; chemicals on the skin should be avoided, and, if necessary, the patient may wear a skin barrier under the appliance for extra protection.

### Conclusions

As chemotherapy becomes more effective against solid tumors, surgeons will employ it more aggressively. Presently available drugs are already effective against many cancers, although surgical resection of local-regional disease is usually required to increase the patient's chance of an ultimate response. As a result, the number of patients who require chemotherapy and have stomas will probably increase. The appropriate aggressive management of the tumor combined with meticulous care of the stoma site can result in very gratifying responses.

## RADIOTHERAPY

Radiotherapy is an integral part of the oncologist's weaponry for combating malignant disease. Over the last three-quarters of a century a wide variety of radiation sources have been developed (cobalt units, linear accelerators, betatrons, radioactive isotopes, etc.) to aid in the selective destruction of cancer cells while leaving sufficient normal cells to maintain functional integrity in the irradiated volume. The cytotoxic action of radiation is mainly caused by damage to cellular deoxyribonucleic acid (DNA) brought about by ionization mechanisms.[9] In general, cells that have been exposed to a lethal radiation dose only die when they begin their next mitotic division, and therefore the rate of cell death in an irradiated cell population depends on the rate at which the cells divide. This accounts for the two phases or radiation effects observed when tissues are irradiated: the acute and the delayed.[3]

The acute radiation reaction is caused by rapid cell death in rapidly dividing tissues such as the skin epidermis or the mucosal epithelium of the gastrointestinal or genitourinary tracts.

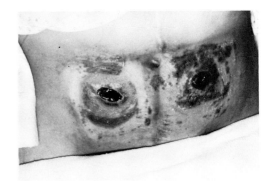

**Figure 8-5.** After surgery creating urinary and bowel diversions, this patient was treated with methotrexate. The peristomal skin became reddened and irritated, even though the appliances did not leak. The reaction disappeared when chemotherapy was completed. (Reprinted with permission from D. B. Rodriguez: Special considerations: Care of the ostomy patient receiving cancer therapy, in D. Broadwell, B. Jackson (Eds): Principles of Ostomy Care, St. Louis, 1982, C. V. Mosby Co.[14])

Consequent to this rapid cell death, an acute inflammatory reaction develops with all its classic features: redness, edema, local heat, and pain. The surface epithelium may slough off at sufficient radiation doses; however, unless exceedingly high-dose irradiation is given, the number of viable cells remaining is always adequate to regenerate the epithelium, and usually within four weeks recovery is nearing completion and the acute inflammation subsides. On a clinical level this acute effect is observed as mucositis, enteritis, or dermatitis. A very severe acute reaction may not heal by fibrosis; this is unusual and should not be confused with a true late-radiation effect.

The late effects of radiation are caused by cell death in slowly dividing cell populations such as arteriolar and capillary endothelial cells. Because these cells normally divide slowly, their death following irradiation occurs correspondingly slowly. Thus, late effects may occur months or years after radiotherapy has been completed. The effects are in large part caused by the slow but progressive necrosis of small blood vessels, leading to ischemia and consequently to fibrosis and, in some instances, to tissue necrosis. The skin may atrophy and lose

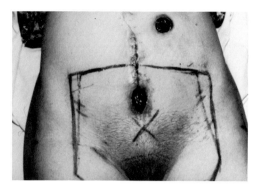

**Figure 8-6.** The treatment field is marked for postoperative irradiation to a patient with a left transverse colostomy and a mucous fistula. Because the mucous fistula stoma was not placed outside the proposed radiation field, it must be watched closely for mucosal reactions. Often, radiation injury causes a mucous fistula to have increased drainage, possibly enough to require a pouch.

well away from the cancerous site. However, an ostomy may overlie a deeper site that does require irradiation. In this circumstance the radiotherapist attempts to devise a radiation field setup that totally avoids the ostomy. The availability of high-energy rotating gantry linear accelerators makes it unlikely that a field will have to include the stoma site incidentally. If radiating through the stoma is unavoidable, the radiotherapist can take certain precautions to minimize the likelihood of complications: (1) use high-energy beams (10–30 MV); (2) use multiple portals of beam entry so that only one traverses the stoma; (3) remove the ostomy pouch during treatments; (4) avoid any metal-containing creams. High-energy x-ray beams have the property of skin sparing, which means that the dose to the skin and subcutaneous tissue (from 0.5 cm to 5 cm deep, depending on the x-ray energy) is lower than the dose to deeper tissues. This effect is lost, however, if an ostomy pouch or heavy metal cream is placed on the skin during the actual irradiation.

its elasticity. The subcutaneous tissues may become fibrotic and indurated. In the intestinal tract, late effects may result in mucosal atrophy, ulceration, fibrosis, stenosis, perforation, or fistula formation. An ostomy irradiated to a high dose may progressively stricture and ultimately close.

In an attempt to reduce the risks of radiation injury and late complications, the radiotherapist must consider a number of factors: the type of radiation beam, the dose delivered, the number of fractions used, the number of days over which radiation will be given, the volume irradiated, and the radiation portal arrangement. It is not within the scope of this book to discuss these complex radiotherapy planning decisions, but we will examine the problems that an ostomy may pose to the radiotherapist and the effects that radiotherapy exerts on ostomy care.

## Problems the Ostomy Poses to the Radiotherapist

The deliberate irradiation of an ostomy to a high dose produces an acute radiation reaction in the surrounding skin and in the stomal mucosa.[6] Fortunately, with the exception of tracheostomies, only rarely does an ostomy require irradiation, since most ostomies are placed

## Effects of Radiotherapy on Ostomy Care

The effects of radiotherapy that most directly affect ostomy care are those related to (1) the skin, (2) stomal-mucosal injury, and (3) gastrointestinal injury. While members of the health care team are preparing patients for radiotherapy treatment, they should carefully explain the effects the treatments may have on the skin, stoma, and bowel.[15]

### Skin Care

The nurse should teach the patient proper skin care around the stoma during radiation treatments (suggestions are summarized in Appendix 8-1). The patient should be cautioned against all forms of irritation to the treatment area. If the peristomal area is within the treatment field, it should be washed gently, using water only and taking care not to remove the treatment-field skin marks (Fig. 8-6). Warm water, gently used around the stoma, usually does not aggravate the area, but vigorous rubbing or toweling must not be done. Cool air is useful in drying the skin, but heat or direct sunlight should be avoided. Soaps, solvents, sprays, ointments, or any of the other ostomy skin preparations should not be applied to the skin without prior approval from the radiotherapist. Some of these preparations contain metals such as zinc or bismuth, which scatter the radiation, increasing the skin dose and the severity of the reaction. For similar reasons, faceplates containing metal or adhesive pouches or tapes containing zinc oxide should not be used during the actual treatment. A simple starch or baby powder may be allowed under the pouch to help absorb the moisture, but we have found a cotton pouch cover preferable; it not only absorbs moisture under the pouch, keeping the area dry, but also provides a soft layer between the appliance and the skin, reducing friction and lessening the risks of mild trauma to the area.

Stool or urine seepage under the faceplate should be meticulously prevented, because the skin is more susceptible to an irritant dermatitis during radiation treatments. The Micropore adhesive is safe and can be used if an adhesive is necessary. Shaving around the stoma is not allowed, since any trauma to the skin can aggravate the reaction.

### Stomal-Mucosal Injury

Gastrointestinal mucosa, because of its rapid cellular division rate, is more radiosensitive than normal skin. Consequently, if the stoma lies within the irradiated field, stomatitis may develop. It is important that the stoma be inspected for mucosal reactions at frequent intervals during therapy. Radiation may cause the stomal mucosa to ulcerate superficially and to exude a layer of fluid. As the exudate coagulates, it forms a whitish membrane on the mucosa, resembling thrush. If the reaction is severe, therapy may have to be discontinued temporarily until the reaction subsides.

When a patient is receiving radiotherapy for active disease at or near the stoma site, the nurse must be sure the appliance opening is large enough to accommodate stomal expansion from tumor growth or edema. Otherwise, the appliance can injure the stoma; we have seen fistulas develop at the stomal skin level as a result of stomal lacerations.

### Gastrointestinal Injury

A patient receiving abdominal or pelvic irradiation may develop diarrhea. If this occurs in a patient who is irrigating his colostomy for regulation, he should stop until the radiation reaction resolves. He can temporarily manage the colostomy with a drainable odor-proof pouch and skin barrier. Adding water to an already liquid stool serves no purpose and only increases bowel irritation. Eating foods that help to control diarrhea, such as bananas, rice, applesauce, and creamy peanut butter, or taking oral medications such as Lomotil may slow the bowel's transit time. Patients with an ileostomy whose ileal output increases may become dehydrated very quickly; they should notify the physician of any such changes in excretion patterns so that fluids and electrolytes can be replaced, intravenously if necessary.

A patient with an external mucous fistula resulting from previous enteric bypass surgery may develop a clear, nonodorous, watery discharge from the mucous fistula as a consequence of irradiation. This is a result of mucositis, and it may or may not subside. The watery drainage may be mistaken for urine. Its volume may be sufficient to require a pouch; if so, we have found that a pediatric urinary pouch is suitable for collecting the drainage.

## HYPERTHERMIA

Since Coley's report in 1893 of 10 patients with malignant disease treated by inducing fever,[5] interest in using hyperthermia as cancer therapy has peaked periodically. When the body temperature is raised above 41°C, the effect is cytocidal. Selective kill of malignant cells occurs within a narrow temperature range, but at temperatures in excess of 41°–42°C, both normal and tumor cells are killed rapidly.[2] Recently, hyperthermia has been evaluated as both a primary and an adjuvant method for treating cancer.[8] Stehlin and associates[16] have used hyperthermic perfusion for patients with melanoma of the extremities, and Pettigrew and associates[13] have reported the clinical effects of whole-body hyperthermia in patients with various advanced malignancies. In addition, the tumoricidal effects of radiation or cytotoxic drugs appear to be potentiated when these treatments are combined with hyperthermia. Currently, methods of inducing hyperthermia include microwaves, radio waves, and ultrasound applied locally or to the whole body.

## Enterostomy Care

Because hyperthermia is most often used in patients who have advanced disease that has not responded to more conventional therapy, the patients treated frequently have undergone previous ostomy surgery to correct urinary or bowel obstructions. Hyperthermia can affect the normal tissues adjacent to the treated tumor, but when hyperthermia is localized, skin problems can usually be avoided by cooling the skin during the treatment.[7,12] If the skin is left unprotected, thermal injury may produce desquamation, erythema, blistering, and ulceration.[10] If the injury occurs around a stoma, care of the area is complicated by the stomal drainage and the need for an appliance. Careful cleansing and the application of a skin barrier under the appliance may be sufficient for recovery when the injury is superficial. If the injury is severe, however, and accompanied by ulceration or necrosis, surgical debridement, skin grafting, or both may be necessary. Enteric mucosa, too, is sensitive to heat therapy,[10] and the stoma should be observed for edema, ulcerations, and necrosis during and immediately after hyperthermia.

## SUMMARY

Patients with ostomies pose challenges to both the medical oncologist and to the radiotherapist, but the presence of an ostomy should not deter them from delivering maximal therapy. Experience has shown that when the problems posed by the ostomy are appreciated, full-dose therapy can be given without placing the patient at any greater risk. Although the side effects of therapy place additional burdens on patients and the members of the health team helping to care for ostomies, a fundamental understanding of the interrelationships between the ostomy and the therapy can obviate many of the problems posed by the cancer treatments.

## APPENDIX 8-1

### Instructions for Peristomal Skin Care During Irradiation

1. If the peristomal area is within the treatment field, wash it gently with water only. Do not remove the treatment-area skin marks.
2. Avoid rubbing or friction. Pat the area dry gently.
3. Cool air may be used to dry the skin, but avoid heat or direct sunshine.
4. Do not use soaps, solvents, sprays, ointments, or any other ostomy skin preparations without specific orders from the radiotherapist.
5. Do not shave around the stoma during irradiation, since any trauma to the skin aggravates the reaction.
6. Do not use dusting or talcum powders during treatments. Some of the powders contain metals such as zinc or bismuth that will further increase the skin dose. A simple starch or baby powder may be used under the pouch to help absorb the moisture. A better suggestion is to wear a cotton pouch cover to absorb the moisture under the pouch, keep the skin dry, and reduce friction.
7. Do not use an adhesive pouch or tape containing zinc oxide during treatments. Micropore or paper tapes are allowed.
8. Do not use a faceplate with metal during the treatments because the metal will increase skin dose.
9. Report skin that becomes reddened or has symptoms of itching, burning, or pain to the radiotherapy physician or nurse.

## REFERENCES

1. Adrian RM, Hood AF, Skarin AT: Mucocutaneous reactions to antineoplastic agents. Cancer 30:143–157, 1980
2. Bleehen NM: Radiotherapy, in Chisholm GD, Williams DI (Eds): Foundations of Urology. Chicago, Year Book Medical Publishers, 1982, pp 616–623

3. Bloomer WD, Hellman S: Normal tissue responses to radiation therapy. N Engl J Med 293:80–83, 1975
4. Click C: Special considerations for the ostomy patient: Chemotherapy. Cancer Bull 33:24–26, 1981
5. Coley WB: The treatment of malignant tumors by

repeated inoculation of erysipelas: With a report of ten original cases. Am J Med Sci 105:487–511, 1893

6. Del Regato JA, Spjut HA, Cox D: Ackerman and Del Regato's Cancer. Diagnosis, Treatment and Prognosis. St. Louis, C. V. Mosby, 1985, pp 59–92

7. Dewey WC, Holahan EV: Thermobiology: Rationale for and problems associated with utilizing hyperthermia in radiotherapy of cancer. Cancer Bull 34:200–208, 1982

8. Field SB, Bleehen NM: Hyperthermia in the treatment of cancer. Cancer Treat Rev 6:63–94, 1979

9. Hall EJ: Radiobiology for the Radiologist. Philadelphia, Harper & Row, 1978

10. Hall EJ, Roizin-Towle L: Biological effects of heat. Cancer Res 44(Suppl):4708–4713, 1984

11. Logothetis CJ, Samuels ML, Ogden S, et al: Cyclophosphamide, doxorubicin, and cisplatin chemotherapy for patients with locally advanced urothelial tumors with or without nodal metastases. J Urol 134:460–464, 1985

12. Moore CL: Hyperthermia: A modern experiment in cancer treatment. Oncol Nurs Forum 2(2):31–35, 1984

13. Pettigrew RT, Galt JM, Ludgate CM, Smith AN: Clinical effects of whole body hyperthermia in advanced malignancy. Br Med J 4:679–682, 1974

14. Rodriguez DB: Special considerations: Care of the ostomy patient receiving cancer therapy, in Broadwell D, Jackson B (Eds): Principles of Ostomy Care. St. Louis, C. V. Mosby, 1982, pp 381–389, 432

15. Di Saia PJ, Creasman WT: Complications of disease and therapy in clinical gynecologic oncology. St. Louis, C. V. Mosby, 1984, pp 507–531

16. Stehlin JS, Giovanella B, de Ioply PD, et al: Results of hyperthermia perfusion for melanoma of the extremities. Surg Gynecol Obstet 140:339–348, 1975

Stephen L. Huber

# 9

# Medications and the Patient with an Ostomy

Patients who have both cancer and an ostomy receive medications for the treatment of their underlying cancer as well as for other coexisting medical conditions. The decisions involved in prescribing drug therapy are more complex, however, when patients have ostomies because of the potential for altered absorption of oral medications and the increased risk of drug-induced complications. Before initiating drug therapy, a practitioner should consider the ostomy type (ileostomy, colostomy, urostomy), the pharmacologic actions of the medication, and the dosage formulation of the drug. Physicians who prescribe drug therapy, pharmacists who dispense the medications, and nurses who administer the drugs should be aware of the particular drugs and product formulations that may cause problems when patients have ostomies. Effective screening of drug orders will minimize ineffective therapy and drug-induced complications. Likewise, educational programs to increase patient awareness of potential problems with medications will result in fewer medication-related complications.

## DRUG ABSORPTION

Unless drugs are administered intravenously, absorption is a prerequisite for drugs to reach their active sites within the various body tissues. Therapeutic activity depends on the concentration of drug at the site of action.

Because drug absorption is a complex process, several factors can influence both the rate and extent of absorption. Tablets and capsules must dissolve prior to absorption; consequently, product formulations that dissolve readily are more rapidly and at times more completely absorbed. Because the majority of drugs are absorbed in the proximal segment of the small intestine, the rate of gastric emptying and the intestinal transit time are important. Gastric emptying and intestinal transit time determine the period of time the drug is in contact with the mucosal surface of the intestine and thereby available for absorption.

In a patient with an ostomy, the intestinal surface area available for drug absorption may be decreased. Gastric emptying, intestinal transit time, pH of the luminal fluid, and mesenteric blood flow may have been altered by the pathologic process that necessitated the formation of the ostomy or by the surgical procedure itself. Consequently, when patients have an ileostomy or a colostomy, the clinician should select product formulations that are rapidly and completely absorbed. Liquid formulations are particularly good for the patient with an ostomy, since they are absorbed rapidly. Although capsules and tablets have not caused documented absorption problems in patients with ostomies, there are no studies in the literature that were designed to look at such problems.

A number of coatings have been developed for a variety of purposes: to mask the taste of certain drugs (sugar coating); to protect acid-labile drugs from the acid environment of the stomach (enteric coating); and to sustain the action of a medication by slowly releasing the active ingredients (sustained-release coating).

THE CANCER PATIENT WITH AN OSTOMY
ISBN 0-8089-1807-9

133

**Table 9-1**
Potential Drug-Induced Problems in Patients with an Ileostomy,
Colostomy, or Urostomy

| Ostomy Type | Drug-Induced Problem | Causative Drug |
|---|---|---|
| Ileostomy | Diarrhea (electrolyte depletion, dehydration) | Laxatives (bisacodyl, senna, phenolphthalein, etc.) |
| | | Antibiotics (clindamycin, lincomycin, penicillins, cephalosporins, tetracyclines, co-trimoxazole, etc.) |
| | | Antacids (magnesium-containing, e.g., Maalox, Mylanta) |
| | | Miscellaneous (colchicine, neomycin, digoxin, cholestyramine) |
| | Diuresis (electrolyte depletion, dehydration) | Diuretics (hydrochlorothiazide, furosemide, chlorthalidone, etc.) |
| Colostomy | Constipation | Antacids (aluminum-containing, e.g., Amphojel, and calcium-containing, e.g., Tums) |
| | | Narcotics (morphine, Levo-Dromoran, codeine, dihydromorphone, oxycodone, etc.) |
| Urostomy | Urinary stone formation | Calcium-containing antacids, sulfa drugs in an acid urine |
| | Diuresis (mechanical) | Diuretics (hydrochlorothiazide, furosemide, chlorthalidone, etc.) |

Coatings are not the only mechanism used to slow absorption: several new systems have been developed that incorporate the drug into a wax matrix that gradually releases the active component into the bloodstream. Following the release of the drug, the expended wax tablet matrix, which is not absorbed, may be detected in the stool or in the ostomy bag. Sustained-release products of all kinds have increased in number due to the convenience of taking fewer doses per day and the improved patient compliance with the prescribed regimen. However, patients with ileostomies or colostomies should avoid sustained-release products; since they are designed to release the drug slowly, they often require absorption along the entire intestinal tract.

Following is a list of the terms currently used to designate sustained-released preparations.

| | |
|---|---|
| Sequels | Tempules |
| Timesules | Plateau Caps |
| Spacetabs | Timespan |
| Chronosule | LA |
| Gradumet | SA |
| MS Contin | SR |
| Spansules | RA |
| Dura-Tab | CR |
| Lon-Tab | Extentabs |

One of these terms usually follows the trade name of the medication.

## DRUG-INDUCED PROBLEMS

Accurate figures on the incidence of drug-induced problems are not available, largely owing to the lack of documentation and reporting. Drug-induced problems in patients with ostomies depend on (1) the pharmacologic actions of the drug and (2) the type of ostomy (Table 9-1).

### Problems Related to Ostomy Type

*Ileostomy*

Patients with ileostomies are particularly vulnerable to drugs that can induce electrolyte depletion and dehydration. Laxatives are one type: they cause diarrhea as an extension of their desired therapeutic effect. Hospitals routinely use such laxatives as bisacodyl to empty the bowel prior to x-ray procedures. However, patients with ileostomies should never use laxatives, either by choice or because of routine procedures.

Antibiotics are frequently prescribed for immunocompromised cancer patients as well as for patients with other infectious diseases. Antibiotics are intended to kill bacteria, but their effect on the bacterial organisms in the gastrointestinal tract may induce diarrhea. Those antibiotics with a broad spectrum of activity, such as tetracyclines, some penicillins, and the second- and third-generation cephalosporins, carry an increased potential for inducing diarrhea. Antibiotics should not be withheld when a patient with an ileostomy has evidence of infection, but their indiscriminate use should be discouraged.

Antacids containing magnesium can cause diarrhea in a patient who has an ileostomy. In addition, certain chemotherapeutic agents commonly used to treat pelvic malignancies (cancers of the bladder, colon, uterus, ovary, and prostate) can induce diarrhea. The incidence of chemotherapy-induced diarrhea appears to be the highest with Adriamycin, 5-fluorouracil, and methotrexate.

Electrolyte depletion and dehydration can also be caused by drugs that induce diuresis and significant amounts of vomiting. Diuretics such as hydrochlorothiazide and furosemide are widely prescribed for many medical conditions, including congestive heart failure and hypertension. Therefore, physicians and patients should be aware of diuretics' potential to induce problems, so as to anticipate them and lessen their impact. Electrolyte imbalance and dehydration secondary to chemotherapy-induced vomiting is most likely with Adriamycin, cyclophosphamide, dacarbazine, 5-fluorouracil, cisplatin, mithramycin, mechlorethamine, and the nitrosoureas (BCNU, CCNU, MeCCNU). Nausea and vomiting usually begin about three to four hours after drug administration and last a few hours. However, in some persons the vomiting is prolonged and can extend up to 24 hours. Antiemetic drugs should be administered prophylactically, and the electrolyte balance and hydration status should be monitored carefully in all patients with an ileostomy.

*Colostomy*

Patients with a colostomy are vulnerable to drug-induced constipation. Antacids containing aluminum or calcium as the primary constituent are common causes of constipation. Narcotic drugs such as codeine, morphine, Levo-Dromoran, dihydromorphone, and others are widely prescribed for pain therapy in cancer patients, including those with colostomies. All of these agents are known to induce a dose-related constipation that is difficult to reverse once it occurs. Again, certain chemotherapy drugs can be the cause of drug-induced problems; for example, the vinca alkaloids (vincristine, vinblastine) have been associated with constipation.

*Urostomy*

A patient who has a urostomy should be aware of drugs that may lead to urinary stone formation. If a patient is prone to forming calcium stones, the amount of calcium contained in some antacid products may be contributory. Sulfa drugs, which are commonly prescribed for urinary tract infections, may crystallize in an acidic urine. Many patients with urostomies routinely acidify their urine by taking vitamin C tablets to decrease odor. In these patients, therefore, the potential for crystallization of the sulfa drug is greatly enhanced.

Diuresis can also adversely affect the patient with a urostomy, but in this instance the problem is mechanical in nature, i.e., the appliance has to be emptied frequently. Potent diuretics, such as furosemide, can cause significant diuresis that may last up to six hours. Cyclophosphamide and cisplatin, chemotherapeutic agents, often require hydration and forced diuresis as part of their administration protocol; this can also pose mechanical problems for patients.

**Problems Common to All**

Some adverse drug reactions can cause serious problems for patients with all types of ostomies. Of these reactions, the dermatologic and myelosuppressive types appear to present the greatest risk to patients with cancer and an ostomy. Adverse reactions affect the skin more than any other site. Dermatologic reactions can lead to excoriation of the skin surrounding the stoma. Consequently, infections and problems in fitting the ostomy appliance may develop.

**Table 9-2**
Drugs That May Discolor Urine

| Drug | Color |
|------|-------|
| Amitriptyline | Blue-green |
| Cascara | Yellow-red |
| Chloroquine | Rust-yellow to brown |
| Chlorzoxazone | Orange to purple-red |
| Danthron | Pink to red |
| Doan's Kidney Pills | Greenish blue |
| Iron | Black |
| Indomethacin | Green |
| Levodopa | Dark on standing |
| Methocarbamol | Dark brown, black, or green on standing |
| Methyldopa | Red to black on standing |
| Methylene blue | Blue-green |
| Metronidazole | Dark brown |
| Nitrofurantoin | Rust-yellow to brown |
| Phenazopyridine | Orange to red |
| Phenolphthalein | Red to yellow-brown |
| Phenothiazines | Pink to reddish-brown |
| Phenytoin | Pink to red to brown |
| Quinacrine | Yellow |
| Quinine | Brown to black |
| Rifampin | Red to orange |
| Senna | Yellow to red |
| Sulfasalazine | Orange-yellow (alkaline urine) |

**Table 9-3**
Drugs That May Discolor Feces

| Drug | Color |
|------|-------|
| Aluminum antacids | White or speckled |
| Antibiotics (oral) | Greenish gray |
| Bismuth | Black |
| Charcoal | Black |
| Iron | Black |
| Indomethacin | Green |
| Phenazopyridine | Orange-red |
| Phenolphthalein | Red |
| Pyrvinium pamoate | Red |
| Anthraquinone laxatives (senna) | Yellow-green to brown |

Penicillins are frequently implicated, but other drugs may also induce skin eruptions. These include barbiturates, bromides, gold salts, phenytoin, iodides, allopurinol, hydralazine, cephalosporins, quinine, salicylates, streptomycin, sulfonamides, thiouracil, and actinomycin D.

Some chemotherapeutic agents cause stomatitis rather than an allergic type of skin reaction as a result of their pharmacologic properties. The stomatitis may occur on a stoma when patients receive methotrexate, actinomycin D, Adriamycin, or cyclophosphamide. The area may be painful and tender to the touch, but there is no specific treatment; the ulcerations heal as the systemic stomatitis is resolved. Soap, solvents, or irritating substances should be avoided in the peristomal area. Patients with a colostomy who normally irrigate for regulation should be instructed to stop irrigations until the stomatitis resolves.

Myelosuppression is a predictable reaction that occurs with many chemotherapeutic agents. Anemia, leukopenia, and thrombocytopenia may occur, and patients may develop petechiae and infectious disease symptoms. The nadir of the white blood cell depression usually occurs seven to ten days after the first day of drug administration. With some chemotherapy (nitrosoureas, mitomycin), the nadir for the white blood cells may be delayed from four to six weeks after the drug is given.

Drug-induced discoloration of the urine (Table 9-2) and feces (Table 9-3) can also occur with numerous drugs and can alarm patients who are not forewarned. Although the direct effect of this discoloration is not usually serious, patients may discontinue drug therapy because of it and this can have important therapeutic consequences. In addition, the discolored urine or feces may permanently stain ostomy appliances.

## DRUGS FOR ODOR CONTROL

Fecal odor may be controlled by internal or external deodorizers. Internal deodorizers are taken by mouth and include chlorophyll, bismuth, and charcoal. Chlorophyll (Derifil) is administered in a dose of one tablet (100 mg) three times daily after meals. The effect is cumulative and may take up to seven days to manifest itself. Patients should be warned of the mild laxative effect and the tendency of the feces to turn a greenish color.

Bismuth subgallate (Devrom) is a useful internal deodorizer prescribed in a dose of one tablet (200 mg) three times daily after meals.

**Table 9-4**
Screening for Drug-Induced Problems in Patients with Ostomies

| | Ostomy Screens | |
|---|---|---|
| I<br>Prescribing | II<br>Dispensing | III<br>Drug Administration |
| Indication for use | Drug vs. indication | Route of administration |
| Benefit vs. risk | Allergy history | Adverse drug reactions |
| Dosage regimen | Route of administration | Response to therapy |
| Therapeutic endpoints | Product formulation | |
| | Drug level monitor | |

Patients may experience a coating and darkening of the tongue. Bismuth interferes with x-ray procedures of the gastrointestinal tract and should be discontinued prior to such procedures.

Several commercial products are available as external deodorizers to be placed directly into the appliance, such as Banish liquid, Fresh Tabs tablets, and Ostobon powder. Listerine and other mouthwash preparations have also been added to the bag to control odor. Aspirin, two tablets crushed and dissolved in the discharge fluid, has also been used; however, it is currently not recommended because of the potential mucosal irritation that can occur when aspirin comes in contact with the skin.

Patients with urinary diversions attempt to control odor by acidifying the urine and drinking sufficient liquid to ensure a dilute urine. Acidic urine inhibits the growth of microorganisms, resulting in less odor. Cranberry juice may be effective in acidifying the urine if 240 ml or more is ingested daily. Vitamin C, 1 gm four times daily, has also been used as a urinary acidifier. Patients should attempt to maintain a urinary pH of about 6.5; to monitor pH, they should test the urine periodically with nitrazine paper.

## SCREENING FOR DRUG-INDUCED COMPLICATIONS

At UT M. D. Anderson Hospital we have found that a screening process to detect and prevent drug-induced complications in patients with ostomies can be an effective quality-assurance tool (Table 9-4). This process should screen the prescribing, dispensing, and administration components of the drug therapy and answer key questions concerning the decisions that are made by the physician, the pharmacist, and the nurse.

The first Ostomy Screen is applied to the prescribing decisions made by the physician. Specifically, a physician should consider the indication for use of all prescribed drug therapy. Classifying the therapy as curative, symptomatic, or prophylactic, and comparing the indication for use to the toxicities that are known for a particular agent, allows a benefit-to-risk assessment to take place. In addition, the physician should exercise care in selecting the route of administration, the specific drug product formulation, and the dosage. Dosage should be individualized to account for differences in body size, drug metabolism and excretion, and other patient characteristics such as the presence of an ostomy. Medications that must maintain blood levels within a narrow therapeutic range (cardiovascular agents, antiepileptic drugs, antibiotics, bronchodilators, etc.) must be carefully monitored in patients with an ostomy. Clinicians should always determine a therapeutic endpoint to allow them to measure the effects of a drug and to guide them in determining when to discontinue or alter therapy.

The second Ostomy Screen is applied to the dispensing process, and particularly to the pharmacist. The pharmacist who reviews the order should use the information on a patient's profile to answer the following questions: (1) What is the indication for each of the drugs ordered? (2) Does the patient have a history of allergic reactions to medications? (3) Are any of the drugs ordered sustained-release preparations? (4) Is the dosage regimen optimal for this patient? (5) Should blood levels of this drug be monitored? If drugs are ordered without any clearly evident indication, the pharmacist should consult the physician to ensure that no unnecessary medications are administered to a patient with an ostomy. If patients are allergic to drugs, the pharmacist should obtain information about the type of reaction, the date, and other descriptive data available. All sustained-release preparations should be avoided, as previously stated, when patients have ileostomies and colostomies. All doses ordered should be compared to the usual ranges, the patient's weight or body surface area, and other patient factors that may alter dosing requirements such as age, renal function, liver function, prior radiation therapy to the bowel, and the type of ostomy a patient has. In general, drugs with a narrow therapeutic range (small differences between therapeutic doses and toxic doses) should be monitored closely. Examples of these drugs are aminoglycoside antibiotics, theophylline compounds, procainamide, quinidine and other antiarrhythmics, and cardiac drugs like digoxin. Digoxin absorption from the intestine is significantly impaired by previous radiation that included the gut area.

The third Ostomy Screen focuses on the process of administering the drugs to patients and monitoring the response to therapy. The nurse should review medications before administering them to ensure that no sustained-release formulations are given to a patient with an ileostomy or colostomy. Adverse drug reactions (ADRs) should be prevented; however, if an ADR is suspected, the nurse should make a written evaluation and document the reaction. If a patient is not responding as expected, then perhaps the drugs are not being absorbed because of the ostomy, and the dose may need to be altered or an alternative therapy selected.

## PATIENT EDUCATION AND COUNSELING

Patients with ostomies should be aware of the potential side effects and drug-induced complications that medications can cause, particularly the medications they are currently taking or are likely to need in the future. Patients should be taught the proper action to take if they suspect a drug-induced problem. In general, for reactions that are not life-threatening, patients should have the following information available when they call their physician or pharmacist concerning a suspected drug-induced problem:

1. The name of the medication (trade name or generic name).
2. The length of time between taking the drug and the first appearance of the problem.
3. What made the reaction better or worse?
4. Have you ever had a similar reaction?

Patients with ostomies should be counseled to avoid or to discontinue using home remedies or self-medication with nonprescription drugs unless their physician has specifically approved the medicine. Routine use of laxatives, antacids, analgesics, and other common nonprescription items can cause serious problems in the ostomate.

Owing to the increase in generic prescribing and the passage of generic-substitution laws in many states, the potential for changes in products dispensed to patients has increased. Patients with ostomies should not change drug brands without consulting their physician or pharmacist about the true "equivalency" of the drugs.

## CONCLUSION

Patients with ostomies are not spared the adverse reactions that medications cause. It takes the efforts of all those who contribute to the care of these patients, including the patients themselves, to prevent drug-induced complications. Optimal drug therapy can be assured through effective screening of the drug prescribing, dispensing, and administration processes to decrease the predictable problems with absorption and side effects.

Stephen B. Tucker
Dorothy B. Smith

# 10

# Dermatologic Conditions Complicating Ostomy Care

A basic clinical knowledge of the structure and function of the skin is important for ostomy care. Most patients are required to use skin adhesives continuously to secure their ostomy appliance. An unhealthy skin surrounding the ostomy site not only makes replacing the appliances painful but also may cause diminished adhesion of the various collecting bags, leading to further leaks and a vicious cycle of ever-increasing irritation.

Cutaneous problems around ostomies have been dramatically reduced since the formation of the specialty of enterostomal therapy. Although ostomy societies began in the late 1960s and early 1970s to collect and disseminate information about ostomy care, skin problems were still being seen in the late 1970s. A report in 1977 indicated that 40 out of 47 patients studied had irritated or ulcerated skin at the site of the ostomy. Ten of those studied knew nothing about protecting the skin surrounding the ostomy, and all 10 of them suffered from severe cutaneous problems.[12]

Enterostomal therapists have reduced this tremendously high rate of cutaneous complications by providing more informed patient care and by encouraging manufacturers to develop better ostomy equipment. Well-designed appliances and less irritating glues and adhesives have been the result. Enterostomal therapy is a fairly new specialty, however. Although its practitioners are constantly learning new and better ways of managing cutaneous conditions

associated with ostomies, large-scale prospective studies comparing methods of skin care have been difficult to perform, and accurate information about cutaneous problems is scant. Nevertheless, the experience of these authors indicates that dermatitis is no longer seen in the majority of ostomy patients, but can be a very severe problem for a minority.

Healthy skin can make the difference between an appliance that seals securely and one that leaks. The peristomal skin retains the general three-level architecture characteristic of skin elsewhere (Fig. 10-1), although with minor modifications. The upper level, the epidermis, is the major cutaneous barrier against physical and immunologic insults. Its surface layer, the stratum corneum, is made up of a stacking of dead cells called corneocytes. These corneocytes are held in place by a highly lipid substance, a sort of intercellular cement, that allows the dead cells to act as a physical barrier to water-based substances. The lipid-corneocyte layer also permits material to be applied to and removed from the surface of the skin without disrupting living cells. Below the corneocytes, the epidermis contains Langerhans' cells, epidermal macrophages that are capable of ingesting potential antigenic compounds to be transferred to lymph nodes. A substance ingested by these cells can ultimately lead to an allergic reaction. The epidermis is a rapidly proliferating tissue: cells take approximately six weeks to progress from the basal, or germinative, layer to the upper layer. This con-

THE CANCER PATIENT WITH AN OSTOMY
ISBN 0-8089-1807-9

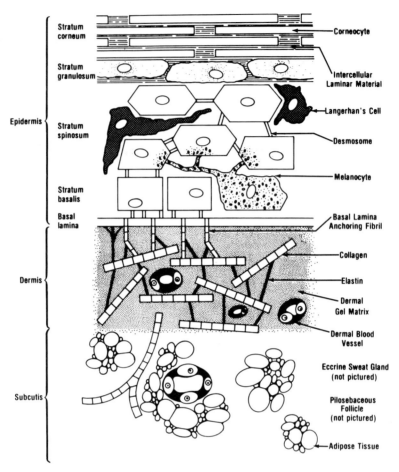

**Figure 10-1.** General architecture of the skin. (Reprinted with permission from S. Tucker, M. Key: Occupational skin disease, in W. M. Rom (Ed): Environmental and Occupational Medicines, Boston, Little, Brown, 1983, p. 301.[24])

stant turnover produces a continuous replacement of cells and a constant refurbishing of the top layer of dead cells.

The middle layer, the dermis, contains numerous components that feed nutrients to the epidermis and provide tremendous strength and stretchability to the skin. The subcutis—the lowest layer of skin—contains fat cells and functions both as an insulation, allowing the temperature on the interior of the body to be quite different from that on the exterior of the body, and as a protective barrier.

The lipid material secreted onto the surface of the skin, together with the action of bacteria, forms a slightly acid pH. This prevents colonization by many pathogenic organisms on the skin. However, in moist areas such as those around ostomy sites, pathogens find a much less hostile environment. The epidermal barrier there is less effective in preventing pathogenic colonization, and substances can more easily penetrate the moist stratum corneum. Nevertheless, the skin surrounding a stoma still has all of the protective mechanisms described above.

## PRESURGICAL CONSIDERATIONS

When surgery to create an ostomy is anticipated, the condition of the skin should be carefully assessed. Evaluation begins with a careful history so as to predict possible reactions to adhesives. Many people describe a history of allergies to Band-Aids and other adhesive patches. This does not necessarily rule out using adhesives with ostomies, because most ostomy adhesives have been screened to eliminate most irritating agents. Potential ostomy adhesives can be patch-tested by applying small pieces of these agents to the arm or the back for 48 hours (Fig. 10-2). If the patient is severely allergic to one of these compounds, the allergy usually shows up. However, one should remember that the skin around the ostomy will be more moist, will undergo repeated application and removal of adhesives, and must tolerate contact with effluent. Therefore, a negative presurgical patch test does not guarantee a trouble-free course with appliance adhesives.

Any preexisting skin diseases should be identified. Several different cutaneous diseases may be triggered at sites of injury such as a stoma site. The most common of these is psoriasis, manifested by a localization of psoriatic lesions at the site of injury. Other conditions include lichen planus, atopic dermatitis, and various immune-complex-associated skin disorders. These skin diseases are not contraindications to an ostomy, but their presence or a history of their presence suggests the potential for problems. It is better to have a plan for prevention or therapy than to be abruptly presented with the complication.

Since no prospective studies have been performed, dermatologists are not sure which dermatoses will cause the greatest difficulties for peristomal skin. For example, the incidence of contact dermatitis is much greater in atopic persons than in those not atopic, and therefore one would expect them to have a greater problem with peristomal dermatitis. An atopic person is more easily sensitized to common allergens causing IgE-mediated hypersensitivity reactions than is the population as a whole. These persons have problems with pruritis when they wear wool clothing and tend to have more cutaneous infections because of increased colonization of pathogens on the skin. They also have a problem with dry skin during the winter. They are much more prone to irritant reactions and therefore would be expected to have more peristomal skin problems. The physician or nurse must consider these factors, and accordingly be especially diligent in providing the least

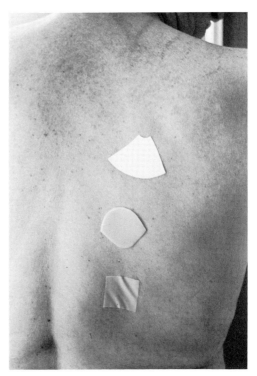

**Figure 10-2.** Applying several patches of ostomy adhesives to the back of a patient with known allergies is part of the preoperative skin assessment.

irritating postsurgical care for an atopic patient. When patients have actual skin lesions at the proposed site of the ostomy, the dermatosis should be treated before surgery to provide the healthiest possible skin around the new ostomy.

## POSTSURGICAL CONSIDERATIONS

When an ostomy is created, numerous small ulcerations occur between the stomal mucosa and the skin that heal by epithelialization. The objectives of immediate postsurgical ostomy care are to create a favorable environment for healing these ulcerations and to prevent further skin breakdown around the stomal incision. A study of ostomy patients with skin erosions and ulcers showed that 51 out of 59 healed rapidly when a properly fitting skin barrier was applied and maintained.[1] If leakage is prevented, the skin can regenerate itself.

The marked swelling at the stoma site is always a problem immediately after surgery. The edema subsides naturally, and as it does, the skin barrier and pouch should be refitted to secure proper skin protection. It is important to measure the stoma on a regular basis to maintain the proper fit between opening and appliance.

The nurse or ET who changes the appliance must learn how to remove adhesive from the skin without causing damage. The trick is to push the skin gently away from the adhesive rather than pull the adhesive off the skin. A warm moist gauze, sponge, or washcloth helps to loosen the adhesive. Any adhesive remaining on the skin after the appliance has been removed can be rolled off gently with a dry gauze or washcloth; excessive rubbing or defatting of the skin around the ostomy injures the epithelium itself.

Solvents and detergents should not be used. In the past they were recommended to clean the skin, but they are not necessary and cause injury. Detergents, solvents, and defatting agents remove the skin's natural defense, the surface film composed of sebum, perspiration, and substances from the stratum corneum. Once this surface film has been removed, several hours are required to build it up again.[10] Detergents or solvents used repeatedly also remove the water-binding substances in the skin that are essential to keep it pliable; the result is dry skin that cracks easily. To replace these water-binding substances requires three to four weeks.[10] Prevention of skin problems requires, therefore, that these substances not be removed.

Although solvents should be kept away from the skin, they can be used to clean reusable faceplates. The patient must allow adequate time for the solvent to evaporate, however, before reapplying the faceplate.

Once the appliance and adhesive have been removed, the nurse should gently wash the skin with warm water, dry it thoroughly by patting it with a cloth or gauze, and apply a clean properly fitted appliance. The appliance can remain in place five to seven days unless there are signs of leakage or symptoms of discomfort under the adhesive. However, a study has shown that daily removal of the ostomy appliance, if done properly, causes only slightly more irritation than removing it once a week.[17] The major irritating factor in this study was the adhesive on the appliance itself. Several adhesives were found to cause a tremendous amount of irritation, whether they were removed daily or weekly. The most gentle adhesives caused very little irritation, suggesting that the material used is more important than how often the appliance is changed.

Shaving around the ostomy site can also cause a problem. This occurs almost exclusively in men, and can be prevented by using gentle techniques, such as shaving in the direction of the hair, completely rinsing the shaving cream from the area, and avoiding using heavily scented compounds near the ostomy. By minimizing injury to the skin, the patient has the least possibility of further complications.

Finally, in this postoperative period, continuous contact between plastic bags and skin should be avoided. Allowing the bag itself to rest against skin distant from the ostomy may lead to sweating, maceration, and cutaneous problems. Covering the pouch with a cloth material usually eliminates this potential problem (Fig. 10-3).

## COMMON CUTANEOUS PROBLEMS

If skin problems do occur, it is important to determine their causes. Only when the cause is known can proper corrective measures be employed.

The type of effluent influences the incidence of dermatitis on the surrounding skin. A study of skin problems seen with urinary diversions, ileostomies, and colostomies[17] revealed that the incidence of minor and severe dermatoses was higher with the colostomies and ileostomies than with the urinary diversions. Although a tight fit of the skin barrier reduces the incidence of dermatitis with all types of stomas, not all instances of irritation can be eliminated. Even a close-fitting skin barrier allows some contact of the skin with the effluent.

### Contact Dermatitis

Contact dermatitis is a term used to designate inflammation of the skin caused by contact with an external agent (Fig. 10-4). The contact dermatitis may be of an irritant or an allergic nature.

#### Irritant Contact Dermatitis

The type of dermatitis encountered most often in a patient with an ostomy is irritant contact dermatitis. An irritant contact dermatitis

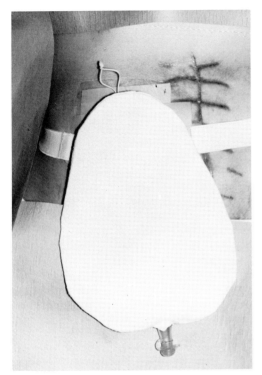

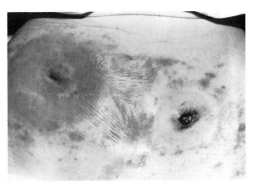

Figure 10-4. After a total pelvic exenteration, this patient's urinary appliance leaked chronically owing to stoma retraction, resulting in erythema and crusting of the skin. The dermatitis is not sharply demarcated on all of the edges but merges gradually into the surrounding skin.

Figure 10-3. A cotton material covering an ostomy pouch absorbs moisture and protects the skin under the pouch. (Reprinted with permission from J Enterostom Ther 8[4]:21, 1981.[19])

is one in which cells sustain a direct toxic injury without developing a specific allergic sensitization. For example, spilling strong acid on the skin causes direct contact injury to the cells. Although we do not recommend using solvents, many patients still use them, and they can cause an irritant contact dermatitis (Fig. 10-5). Fecal products, marked pH changes, and enzymes also cause an irritant dermatitis. Ostomy deodorants have been reported to be causative agents.[8] Unless contact with an irritating substance is constant, irritant reactions usually subside.

Irritant dermatitis develops in two stages. In the first the defense mechanism in the skin is interrupted, increasing the possibilities for harmful substances to penetrate the skin. The injury at this point is localized in the stratum corneum and may be reversible if the irritant is removed from the skin.

The second stage is an eczematous inflam-

mation. The factor that injured the skin at the beginning of the course does not have to be the factor that later maintains the dermatitis. For example, the skin can be injured initially by contact with stool, urine, ileal effluent, or solvents. The injury can then be maintained by something else, such as a detergent.[10] Once a dermatitis has developed, slight physical trauma or even soap and washing can potentiate the injury. If the irritant dermatitis has lasted a long time before treatment is started, it may require months to heal. Even after the skin has healed clinically its defenses are reduced, and it may not tolerate substances such as soaps, deter-

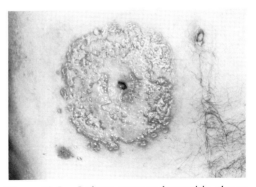

Figure 10-5. Irritant contact dermatitis, the result of using solvent around a urinary stoma to remove adhesive.

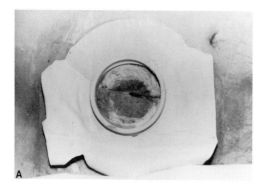

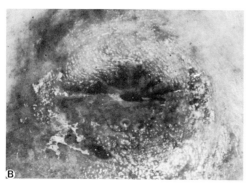

**Figure 10-6.** **A,** the patients' urinary faceplate opening is too large for the stoma opening, leaving skin continually exposed to urine (reprinted with permission from J Enterostom Ther 11[1]:36, 1984[23]). **B,** the faceplate has been removed and the skin cleansed. Note the large area of chronic contact dermatitis resulting from the continued urine contact causing erythema, scaling, and thickening of the epidermis (lichenification).

gents, or solvents that heretofore had no effect.[10]

Irritant dermatitis is erythematous in appearance. It is usually painful, even in its mildest forms. Treatment consists of, first, rinsing the skin well with warm water and drying it thoroughly. A hair dryer set on cool is a good drying agent. Next, if indicated, a skin barrier is applied. The gelatin- and pectin-based barriers adhere to slightly moist skin and allow the skin to heal if stomal drainage is kept away. Finally, a properly fitting appliance is applied.

When the skin at the site is weeping, it should be sealed to prevent the weeping. A useful sealing agent is a modified Burrow's solution, which combines a metal salt with a weak

acid. This also helps control microorganisms. Once the weeping has been controlled, the medications can perform their specified purpose because they are not continually washed off by draining serum.

If a dermatitis is so severe that an appliance will not stick to the skin, then some other form of drainage collection must be employed temporarily. Meanwhile the skin can be treated with the Burrow's solution and with anti-inflammatory agents such as steroids. This treatment usually leads to marked improvement in two or three days, at which time a properly fitting appliance can be placed.

When dermatitis is severe, steroid creams are more useful than steroid ointments. Because the latter contain more oil, they interfere with appliance adhesion and trap moisture, leading to further maceration of the inflamed skin. Steroid creams are not recommended for routine ostomy care, however, because they may cause such unwanted side effects as thinning of the skin, striae, and a propensity to infection.

Physicians and nurses must be aware that strong fluorinated steroids can be used for only a short period of time at the ostomy site. Since any agents that are applied directly to the skin are occluded by adhesives when the appliance is in place, the tendency of topical steroids to cause atrophy and cutaneous infection is exaggerated. Therefore, very strong steroids should never be used; when occluded, the weaker hydrocortisone preparations are very effective. If they are not, one should very strongly suspect allergic contact sensitization. Allergic contact dermatitis of skin repeatedly exposed to allergen presents a recurrent and resistant picture in spite of topical steroid use.

Irritation dermatitis can result not only from externally applied agents but often from stomal drainage. Ileostomy effluent, because of its high enzymatic content and high pH, can severely damage the skin in a short time (see Fig. 3-21A). Urine or feces on the skin may act more slowly, but they too can be irritating. Skin problems from stomal contents have several origins. The most common is a skin irritation that results because the opening in the faceplate or appliance is larger than the stoma, allowing stomal contents to drain out onto the skin (Fig. 10-6). Stomal size and appliance fit should be checked several times during the postoperative period as

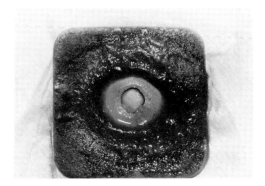

**Figure 10-7.** A skin barrier wafer made of gelatin and pectin was removed from a urinary diversion after 48 hours. The skin barrier has melted, leaving the immediate peristomal skin exposed to urine. This can result in an acute or chronic form of contact dermatitis.

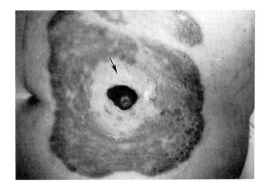

**Figure 10-8.** An allergic contact dermatitis caused by a substance in the adhesive to which the patient has become specifically sensitized. The area has diffuse erythema and crusting. The inner ring around the stoma (arrow) was under a skin barrier and was not in direct contact with the sensitizing agent.

the stomal edema subsides and the stoma shrinks.

Occasionally an appliance opening or faceplate allows urine, stool, or ileal effluent to leak under the adhesive. This can be due to a skin crease, fold, retention suture, or too much back pressure from a full pouch. If the pouch is immediately changed and the skin cleaned, the skin may not become irritated. If the stomal contents are not removed from the skin, however, irritation will occur. It is important to remember, particularly with a urinary diversion, that skin barriers made of karaya, gelatin, or pectin may be slowly absorbed, leaving urine trapped next to the skin. Also some barriers melt in the presence of urine, leaving the skin exposed to a continuous bath of urine (Fig. 10-7). For these reasons we do not recommend applying skin barriers for urinary diversions on a long-term basis.

Irritant dermatitis is reversible, but proper appliance adherence is necessary to reverse it. Once the irritation has progressed to a weeping dermatitis, the damaged skin may be further injured by agents that would not cause a dermatitis on normal, intact skin. Here solvents, particularly, are contraindicated, and detergents may worsen the dermatitis.

*Allergic Contact Dermatitis*

Allergic contact dermatitis presents a picture similar to that of irritant contact dermatitis, including redness and weeping of the peristomal skin (Figs. 10-8 and 10-9). The difference is that a specific immune response has occurred that has sensitized the patient to certain low-molecular-weight chemical agents. With a contact allergy, even very minute exposures to the sensitizing agent provoke a dermatitis. The situation is similar to that of someone who is allergic to poison ivy and then puts just a very tiny amount of poison ivy under the stomal appliance. What occurs is an allergic dermatitis reaction. More often, however, the contact dermatitis is fairly mild because the allergy to the offending substance is low grade (Fig. 10-10). Health care personnel should remember that agents placed on inflamed or open skin like that around an inflamed ostomy site, which has lost its usual barriers, are more likely to cause allergenic sensitization (Fig. 10-11). Once this sensitization occurs, the person can no longer tolerate exposure to even a small amount of the material.

One can perform a patch test for allergic sensitization by using a small piece of the potentially offending agent or by learning the agent's chemical composition and applying the chemicals directly (Fig. 10-12). The latter course is preferred but not always possible, because obtaining even a listing of the ingredients, much less the specific chemicals used, is often difficult. However, patch testing is more effective when one can use a more concentrated form of a test substance. The very low concentration of allergen that is sufficient to cause a reaction in

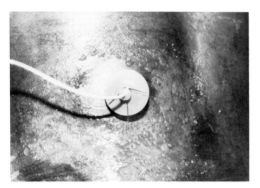

**Figure 10-9.** Allergic contact dermatitis from adhesive tape, showing wet desquamation and blistering around a catheter site.

open peristomal skin is frequently not adequate to provoke an allergic dermatitis in intact arm or back skin, where the testing takes place.

Figure 10-13 illustrates an allergic contact dermatitis that developed after an irritant dermatitis. The allergic dermatitis was caused both

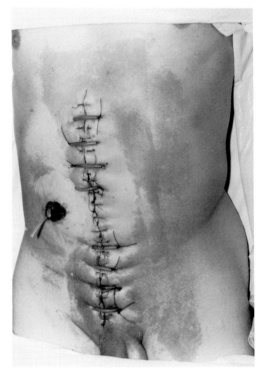

**Figure 10-11.** Allergic dermatitis caused by the tape used to apply a pressure dressing after surgery. The peristomal area was protected by a skin barrier and was not affected.

by the cream applied under the ostomy appliance and by the adhesive itself. In this instance, the patient's skin reacted positively when the adhesive alone was applied in a different spot. We were unable to get the ingredients to patch test this patient, but switching to a totally dif-

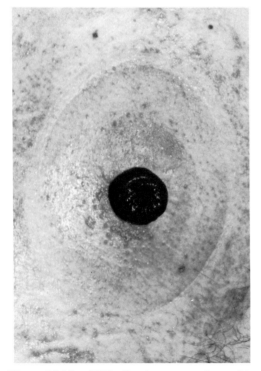

**Figure 10-10.** Mild allergic contact dermatitis under the adhesive of an ileostomy faceplate. Note that the area of mild erythema matches the pattern of the adhesive.

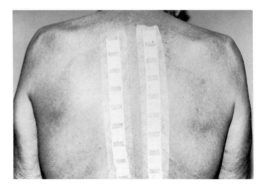

**Figure 10-12.** Small amounts of potentially offending agents applied to a patient's back test for allergic sensitization.

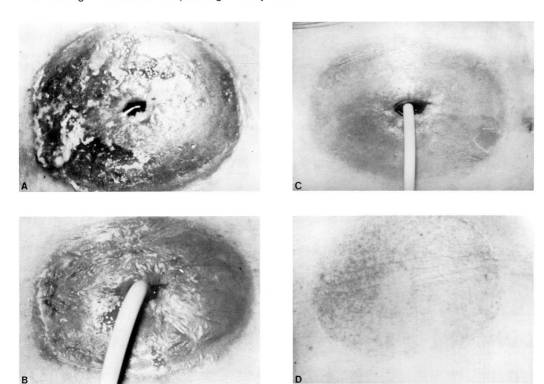

**Figure 10-13.** **A**, a patient with a urinary diversion presented in clinic with a severe contact allergic dermatitis. Note that the sharply demarcated area matches the area of the faceplate's contact with the skin. **B**, the dermatitis was so acute that the patient was hospitalized and the urine diverted by catheter drainage. Removing the sensitizing agent and using Burrow's solution and topical corticosteroid cream immediately improved the lesion. Note the crusting on the skin surface. **C**, the same patient after 12 days of therapy. Note that the epidermis is healing, although it still appears very thin and friable. Oozing and vesicle formations have cleared. **D**, the offending agent was applied to the patient's back as a patch test, resulting in mild dermatitis within 48 hours.

ferent type of adhesive and not using the cream allowed the dermatitis to resolve. The initial dermatitis, nevertheless, was strong enough that hospitalization was required. Burrow's solution and strong corticosteroids were applied to the skin for three weeks while the urine was diverted with a catheter. It is important to realize that once the contact dermatitis is present, not only can it be evoked by a very small amount of the allergen, but also the patient usually remains allergic to that substance for the rest of his or her life.

Substances that are frequently recommended in the ostomy literature to treat dermatitis include antacids and karaya powder. Clinically, these agents have been demonstrated to reverse irritation by providing a nonirritating barrier; the antacids may often neutralize an acid type of effluent from the ostomy drainage. These are not useful, however, when the dermatitis is as severe as that of this patient. For him, topical corticosteroids were the recommended treatment.

### Yeast Infections

*Monilia* infections are very common at ostomy sites. *Candida* species are the most usual infecting organisms, since they typically inhabit the bowel. *Candida* easily establishes itself in a moist environment like that at an ostomy site. Just as damaged skin is susceptible to irritant dermatitis, it is also predisposed to a *Candida* infection (Fig. 10-14). Systemic factors that may

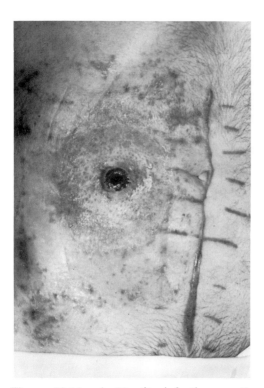

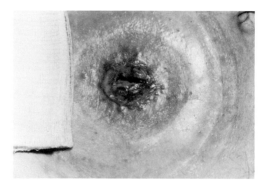

**Figure 10-15.** Hyperplastic growth of the epithelium around an ileostomy. (Reprinted with permission from A. Gunn (Ed): Cancer Rehabilitation, Raven Press, 1984, p. 113.[22])

**Figure 10-14.** A *Monilia* infection on the peristomal skin around a urinary ostomy. The erythematous lesion has small superficial pustules present as satellite lesions along the periphery. (Reprinted with permission from Clin Gastroenterol 11:322, 1982.[20])

add to this predisposition include diabetes mellitus, iron deficiency, cancer, an immune deficiency, myelosuppression from chemotherapy, and iatrogenically induced hypersteroidism. Systemic drugs such as antibiotics, which may decrease the normal bacterial flora, can also predispose skin to *Candida*. A potassium hydroxide mount or culture can provide a positive identification, although the appearance of the peristomal area is often distinct enough for the physician to select appropriate therapy. A *Candida* lesion is characterized by a bright red erythematous center and a surrounding group of red satellite papules. The skin may have a white superficial coating and may itch.

Treatment consists of an anticandidal powder, applied each time the appliance is changed. The powder not only helps to absorb moisture, but also has a specific antipathogenic effect on

yeast organisms. When the infection is severe, it should be treated daily. The skin should be carefully dried before the powder is applied. A plasticized dressing may be applied over the powder; it is often required because the powder interferes with the adhesion of most adhesive agents. Treatment should be continued for several days after the area has clinically cleared. As with any medication that is applied to skin under occlusion, the potential for allergic sensitization is high even with these antimicrobial agents. Therefore, we do not recommend using them prophylactically.

## Hyperplasia

Hyperplasia of the epithelium occurs often around urinary stomas but may also be seen around colostomy and ileostomy stomas (Figs. 10-15 and 10-16). The term *hyperplasia* is used to describe a thickened epithelium that may be either verrucose or smooth. In the latter, the epithelium appears almost normal but is slightly thickened and infringes upon the stomal mucosa, making the junction somewhat obscure. Hyperplasia is a reaction to a low-grade irritant contained in urine or in ileostomy or colostomy effluents. It usually develops after long-standing contact between the irritating agents and the skin, which may be the result of a faceplate with an opening larger than the stoma or a poorly fitting faceplate that allows materials to get under the seal.

The proper treatment of hyperplasia begins

with removing the irritating effluent from the skin by applying a properly fitting appliance. The opening of the appliance should be no more than $\frac{1}{16}$-inch larger than the stoma and should not allow skin to be exposed to drainage. Even though no carefully controlled studies have reported a beneficial effect, some patients try to acidify the urine. Hyperplastic epithelium is usually treated with acid soaks, using vinegar or acetic acid, although it is unclear just how this treatment works. If the hyperplasia is softened, however, it is easier to push back with the appliance faceplate. Using plasticized karaya washers, such as Colly-seel, is another way to soften the keratosis.

## UNUSUAL CUTANEOUS PROBLEMS

### Necrotizing Phycomycosis

Fatal necrotizing phycomycosis infections have been reported to occur at the ostomy site.[26] This problem is unusual in a normal person, but not so rare in a cancer patient with an ostomy. Because many cancer patients have a reduced immune status and because an ostomy site is abnormally occluded, the infectious agents can run a much more virulent course than one normally expects. A biopsy should be performed on any area of persistent or rapidly spreading redness to identify or rule out phycomycosis. This type of severe infection occurs most often in patients with diabetes.

### Cutaneous Amebiasis

A case of cutaneous amebiasis has been reported occurring in a patient with a colostomy.[18] This might be expected, since the amebae are normally bowel organisms. Because the effluent at the ostomy site may contain any organism that infects the bowel or urinary tract, the stoma site must be watched when those organs are infected. Organisms that are not problematic on normal skin can cause infections on altered peristomal skin, and so it is important to investigate any resistant problems, using cultures and histologic techniques as needed.

### Parastomal Varices

A bluish discoloration of the skin around the stoma site that blanches when pressed may indicate parastomal varices, or a caput medu-

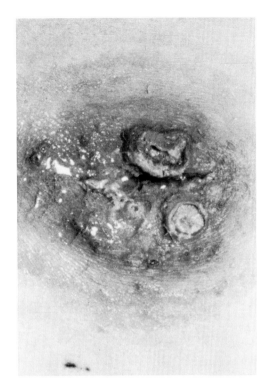

**Figure 10-16.** A severe case of hyperplasia that developed just three months after the patient received a urinary diversion. The skin barrier she had been wearing was melting in urine, leaving her skin continually wet. Note the gray, verrucose (wart-like), hyperkeratotic lesions that have almost occluded the mucosa of the stoma. This form of hyperkeratosis is very painful.

sae.[11,16] This may be seen in patients who have cirrhosis of the liver or metastases to the liver, with corresponding increased portal pressure. In caring for patients with this problem, one should be aware of the possibility of severe hemorrhage at the ostomy site. A pressure dressing may be sufficient, but if it is not, revision of the ostomy site and destruction of the varices at the site may be necessary.

### Recurrent Tumor

Metastatic disease may impact on an ostomy by developing in the adjacent skin (Fig. 10-17) or within the bowel used to construct the

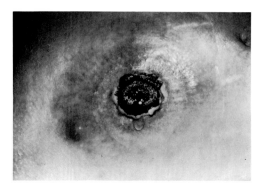

**Figure 10-17.** Recurrent tumor. A cutaneous tumor nodule erupting next to an ileal conduit stoma.

ostomy. The former may cause problems with appliance adherence and the latter may result in obstruction and fistula formation. Although cutaneous metastases occur most often with breast cancer, they have been reported in association with cancers of the large intestine, ovary, and bladder.[2,3,15]

Chemotherapy is usually the treatment of choice, but selected situations may indicate surgical excision, radiotherapy, or both. Successful management of the ostomy appliance frequently requires using skin barriers around the stoma and avoiding hard faceplates. When the malignancy threatens to occlude the lumen of an ileal conduit, an indwelling catheter may be necessary to facilitate urinary drainage.

### Pyoderma Gangraenosum

Pyoderma gangraenosum is another systemic skin lesion that may occur under a faceplate. It may be associated with malignant disorders and is directly related to ulcerative colitis,[25] a disease that carries a high incidence of colon malignancy. Its incidence also increases among patients with myeloma and leukemia.[13]

Lesions that occur under an ostomy faceplate are often not identified correctly and are undertreated. The lesions appear as irregular gangrenous areas with ragged, reddish-purple borders,[4] and may enlarge progressively, tunnel, and extend in a creeping fashion until an ostomy appliance can no longer adhere to the skin. Although measures for keeping the ulcer clean and preventing bacterial overgrowth are helpful,

topical treatment alone is insufficient. It is necessary to treat the cutaneous eruption with large doses of corticosteroids, after making certain the ulcers are not infectious. As this inflammatory process is brought under control, ulcers heal and an appliance can once again be used. This condition should be considered when rapidly advancing cutaneous ulcers occur with various associated bowel and hematopoietic diseases.

### Psoriasis

Psoriasis affects two to four percent of the white population and varies in severity from a few isolated lesions to a widespread dermatosis. The cause remains unknown but a family history is common. The lesions are usually sharply demarcated, nonpruritic, erythematous papules or plaques covered with white scales.[6] The lesions frequently have a symmetrical distribution involving the elbows and knees, as well as the scalp, back, and buttocks. The nails, eyebrows, axilla, umbilicus, and genital region may become involved. Often the disease becomes generalized.

In view of the frequency of psoriasis within the general population, it is not surprising that many patients requiring an ostomy suffer with the disease. Although local trauma is known to precipitate psoriatic eruptions at the local trauma site (Koebner phenomenon), this has not been the problem in the patients we have treated (Fig. 10-18). Treatment follows the same guidelines as those for patients without an ostomy, namely, applying lubricants, keratolytics, and topical tar or corticosteroid preparations. In severe cases, ultraviolet light treatment or even chemotherapeutic agents may be necessary.

### Pemphigus

Pemphigus is a serious, potentially fatal, blistering skin disorder, the result of an autoimmune phenomenon.[7] The disorder is most frequently characterized by bullae developing first in the mouth and later on normal-appearing skin. As the bullae rupture they leave a raw, denuded area that later becomes crusted. Occasionally, the process may resemble exfoliative dermatitis with or without tiny vesicles. This was the situation in one of our patients (Fig. 10-19). Treatment usually requires large doses of corti-

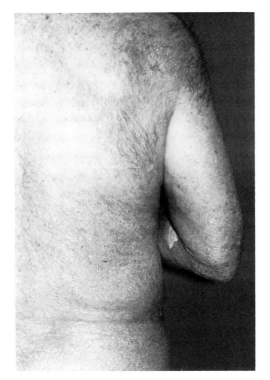

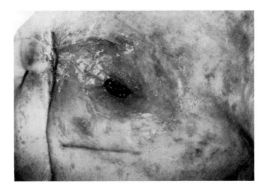

**Figure 10-19.** Peristomal pemphigus in a patient who had a descending colostomy. (Reprinted with permission from J Enterostom Ther 8[5]:32, 1981.[21])

## Mycosis Fungoides

Mycosis fungoides is a cutaneous malignancy categorized as a cutaneous T-cell lymphoma[9] (Fig. 10-20). It presents initially with eczematous plaques and spreads progressively to involve most of the skin and, eventually, lymph nodes and other organs. Patients' average life expectancy ranges from seven to ten years following diagnosis. If the disease is clinically limited to the skin, treatment may include topical chemotherapy, using such drugs as nitrogen mustard, and total-body electron-beam therapy. The malignant cells of mycosis fungoides are radiosensitive, but the problems and toxicity that follow a total-skin x-ray bath can cause

**Figure 10-18.** Psoriasis of the back of a patient with a urinary ostomy for cancer of the bladder. (Reprinted with permission from J Enterostom Ther 8[5]:31, 1981.[21])

costeroids, which stop the blister formation and, over several weeks, lead to healing of the eroded areas.

## Dermatomyositis

Dermatomyositis is an uncommon disease affecting the skin and skeletal muscles. The incidence of associated internal malignancy in adults with this disease is significant.[5] The cutaneous lesions consist of edematous erythematous patches that extend gradually until they involve large areas of the skin.[14] Involvement of the skeletal muscles causes progressive weakness, muscular pain, and atrophy.

The authors have seen one patient with dermatomyositis whose skin was very hard and dry. We used a soft two-piece wafer appliance, even though we recognized that the wafer would melt with the urine and require frequent changes. A hard plate was not suitable because it tended to rock on the patient's firm abdomen.

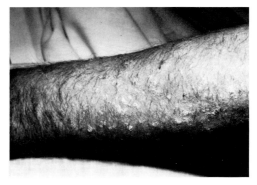

**Figure 10-20.** Mycosis fungoides developed as eczematous plaques on the skin. This patient also has cancer of the bladder and has been treated by cystectomy and urinary diversion.

severe complications such as agranulocytosis, radiation dermatitis, and even death. Nearly all patients receiving total-body electron-beam therapy experience severe dryness of the skin and various degrees of scaling. A few patients also have erythema, desquamation, or frank bullae.[15]

If a patient with mycosis fungoides needs ostomy surgery, the health care team must determine what type of treatment his abdominal skin has had and what type the parastomal areas will need in the future. Usually treating the generalized cutaneous disease causes sufficient healing of the skin so that ostomy care can proceed routinely.

## CONCLUSION

Preventive measures are the best ways to eliminate cutaneous problems around ostomies. Presurgical evaluation of the patient is very important, not only for proper ostomy placement but also to determine any special measures that may be needed because of preexisting skin problems. The immediate postsurgical period is also a very important time: most patients need intensive ostomy care to cope with heavy drainage and the changing stoma size. Although manufacturers have made significant advances in adhesives and in compounds applied to the skin around an ostomy, the potential for irritant and contact dermatitis and for infections remains. The best way to prevent these problems is to use the least-irritating types of substances at the ostomy site and to follow procedures that minimize physical irritation. Maintaining a properly fitting ostomy appliance then becomes the most important aspect.

If a problem does occur, it should be specifically identified. Infections should be diagnosed and properly treated; dermatitis should be evaluated as irritant or allergic, and steroid treatment applied if necessary. A decrease in weeping from the wound is important for any type of therapy to be effective.

Unusual problems may develop because of the nature of the health of many of the patients. Since complications can be fatal, it is important that any unusual manifestation around the ostomy site be evaluated thoroughly to identify or to rule out infectious or neoplastic problems.

Fortunately, the majority of ostomates have very few skin problems, but health care personnel should be aware of the dangers and the treatments for those whose problems are severe. Prospective studies that evaluate and monitor the types of dermatologic problems that affect ostomates with cancer will, we hope, supply data useful to those who care for these patients.

## REFERENCES

1. Beernaerts A, Bouffioux C, Chantrie M, et al: The management of abdominal wall stomata: Skin protection, peristomal wound healing and support for the collecting bag. A multicenter study. Acta Chir Belg 76:533–537, 1977
2. Brownstein MH, Helwig EB: Metastatic tumors of the skin. Cancer 29:1298–1307, 1972
3. Brownstein MH, Helwig EB: Patterns of cutaneous metastasis. Arch Dermatol 105:862–868, 1972
4. Brunsting LA, Goeckerman WH, O'Leary PA: Pyoderma (ecthyma) gangraenosum: Clinical and experimental observations in five cases occurring in adults. Arch Dermatol 22:655–680, 1930
5. Callen JP, Starviski MA, Voorhees JJ: Cutaneous manifestations of systemic illness, in: Manual of Dermatology. Chicago, Year Book Medical Publishers, 1980, pp 129–161
6. Callen JP, Starviski MA, Voorhees JJ: Papulosquamous disorders, in: Manual of Dermatology.

Chicago, Year Book Medical Publishers, 1980, pp 15–32
7. Callen JP, Starviski MA, Voorhees JJ: Vesicular and bullous disorders, in: Manual of Dermatology. Chicago, Year Book Medical Publishers, 1980, pp 33–52
8. Davis, MG: Contact dermatitis from an ostomy deodorant. Contact Dermatitis 4:11–13, 1978
9. Edelson RL: Cutaneous T-cell lymphoma, in Fitzpatrick TB, Eisen AT, Wolff K, et al (Eds): Update: Dermatology in General Medicine. New York, McGraw Hill, 1983, pp 143–154
10. Fregert S: The skin's defense against chemical and physical agents, in Fregert S (Ed): Manual of Contact Dermatitis. Chicago, Year Book Medical Publishers, 1974, pp 11–39
11. Graeber GM, Ratner MH, Ackerman NB: Massive hemorrhage from ileostomy and colostomy stomas due to mucocutaneous varices in patients

with co-existing cirrhosis. Surgery 79:107–110, 1976

12. Halevy A, Adam Y, Eschar J: Ileostomates in Israel. Dis Colon Rectum 20:482–485, 1977

13. Kolff K, Stingl G: Pyoderma gangraenosum, in Fitzpatrick T, Eisen AZ, Wolff K, et al (Eds): Update: Dermatology in General Medicine. New York, McGraw Hill, 1983, pp 174–183

14. Lever WF, Schaumburg-Lever G: Connective tissue disease, in Lever WF, Schaumburg-Lever G (Eds): Histopathology of the Skin. St. Louis, J. B. Lippincott, 1983, pp 445–471

15. Lever WF, Schaumburg-Lever G: Metastatic carcinoma and carcinoid, in Lever WF, Schaumburg-Lever G (Eds): Histopathology of the Skin. St. Louis, J. B. Lippincott, 1983, pp 590–597

16. Lo RK, Johnson DE, Smith DB: Massive bleeding from an ileal conduit. J Urol 131:114–115, 1984

17. Marks R, Evans E, Clarke TK: The effects on normal skin of adhesives from stoma appliances. Curr Med Res Opin 5:720–725, 1978

18. Polano MK: A case of cutaneous amebiasis. Dermatologica 151:253–256, 1975

19. Rodriguez DB: Radiotherapy and the ostomy patient: Special considerations. J Enterostom Ther 8(4):21–22, 1981

20. Rodriguez DB: Stoma care. Clin Gastroenterol 11(2):318–326, 1982

21. Rodriguez DB: Treatment for three ostomy patients with systemic skin disorders: Psoriasis, pemphigus, and dermatomyositis. J Enterostom Ther 8(5):31–32, 1981

22. Smith DB: Rehabilitation of the ostomy patient, in Gunn A (Ed): Cancer Rehabilitation. New York, Raven Press, 1984, pp 101–120

23. Smith DB, Johnson DE: Stoma complications. J Enterostom Ther 11(1):35–39, 1984

24. Tucker S, Key M: Occupational skin disease, in Rom WM (Ed): Environmental and Occupational Medicine. Boston, Little, Brown, 1983, pp 301–311

25. Williams S: Recognizing peristomal pyoderma gangraenosum. J Enterostom Ther 11(2):77–79, 1984

26. Wilson CB, Siber GR, O'Brien TF, Morgan AP: Phycomycotic gangrenous cellulitis. Arch Surg 111:532–538, 1976

Joseph N. Corriere, Jr.

# 11

# Special Problems in Children

Most urinary diversions and bowel stomas in children are created to correct congenital anomalies or as a consequence of these anomalies. Pelvic tumors that require extirpative surgery of the bladder, rectum, or both in children are usually rhabdomyosarcomas of the bladder, prostate, or vagina; epithelial tumors of the bowel or bladder are extremely rare in children. The rhabdomyosarcomas, which arise from the soft tissues in the pelvis, are highly malignant, tend to involve local structures, and eventually metastasize to distant sites. Before we had effective chemotherapy for children with rhabdomyosarcoma, treatment of these patients was usually unsuccessful. Radical surgery, even when followed by radiation therapy, resulted in few long-term survivors.

Consequently, in 1972 a number of institutions united to form the Intergroup Rhabdomyosarcoma Study. Patients in the study were treated first by surgical ablation of the local tumor—partial or total cystectomy or vaginectomy—followed by radiotherapy and chemotherapy. More recently, physicians have placed greater reliance on primary chemotherapy,[10] suggesting that surgery be limited to biopsy of the lesion and resection of tumor in those patients who respond incompletely to chemotherapy. However, the results have been disappointing. Neither primary intensive chemotherapy alone nor chemotherapy given concurrently with radiotherapy has produced complete tumor responses in most patients.[9] It appears that, to

survive, children with these devastating neoplasms will continue to need extirpative surgery and the creation of urinary and bowel stomas.

Rarely, other pelvic neoplasms necessitate an excision of the bladder, bowel, or rectum to cure or relieve bowel or urinary obstruction. Unfortunately, because of the small stature of the patients and the nature of pelvic tumors to extend locally, many of these patients require both a urinary and a gastrointestinal stoma.

## STOMA SITE SELECTION

Locating the urinary or fecal stoma site in a child requires considerable forethought and attention to detail. The small surface area allows very little margin for error. The stoma must accommodate a collection device and allow the patient to participate in all the normal activities of childhood without fear of urine or stool leakage, which would be especially embarrassing to a vulnerable youngster.

Stoma site selection in a child older than three years is best accomplished by having the patient wear an appliance attached to his skin as a test over a two- or three-day period. During this experimental trial, urinary collection appliances should be filled with water while they are worn. As a theoretical guideline, we place the child supine and draw a triangle from the umbilicus to the anterior superior iliac spine, through the midline of the pubis, and up again to the umbilicus. The middle of the triangle may be the best spot for the stoma. Obviously, scars from previous procedures, skin folds, or creases may change the site.

The child then sits up, and we examine the site to see if it does afford the flattest possible surface on which to glue a collection device. If the child must wear braces, the orthopedic surgeon and braceman should be consulted to be sure that belts from their devices will be compatible with the stoma and the appliance.

The goal is an appliance that adheres to the body for a minimum of three days and three nights, is comfortable in all positions, permits all normal activities, and is easily concealed under normal clothing.

## STOMA CREATION

Stoma creation in a child is really no different from stoma creation in an adult, except that the child's stoma is expected to last many years longer! Because both stoma and bowel grow in proportion to the rest of the body, the diversion should never need to be revised if it is constructed properly and cared for appropriately.

The tension lines of the skin in the abdominal wall run transversely, and therefore incisions made in the direction of tension lines produce less contraction than incisions perpendicular to tension lines.[3,33] In addition, removing triangular or square skin segments rather than the traditional round skin segment causes less long-term contraction of the stoma.[20]

The surgeon must pay strict attention to fixing the bowel segment to the abdominal fascia to prevent peristomal hernias. These are particularly troublesome in patients who have a temporary loop colostomy created for bowel obstruction. Absorbable suture, preferably polyglycolic acid material, should be used to fix the mucosal edge to the skin. Catgut material causes an intense inflammatory reaction, and removing nonabsorbable sutures from a scared, squirming child is very difficult.

Finally, the bud stoma rather than the flush stoma appears to offer the best appliance fit. Although flush stomas are quite acceptable in adults who lead a more sedentary life, bud stomas are most suitable to active and less careful children. The infant, child, or young adult should be encouraged to do all the things

young people do. A well-constructed stoma with a tight-sealing appliance encourages this normal life-style.

## STOMA CARE

Stoma care for children is similar to that for adults with the very important exception that, in the very young, the parents have to provide this service. Some clinicians have suggested that the urinary stoma or colostomy of children younger than three can be managed as satisfactorily with disposable diapers as with an ostomy appliance. However, using diapers creates problems. A child with a urinary diversion passes urine continually onto the skin, while an infant who has a bladder stores and empties urine periodically, although admittedly in an incontinent fashion. A urinary pouch protects the skin, prevents the odor and discomfort that come from being wet, and relieves parents from diaper changes throughout the night (Fig. 11-1). An ileostomy in a small child certainly should never be managed with a diaper, since the enzymes in the effluent can rapidly cause a severe dermatitis (see Chapter 10).

In addition, and most important, stoma care started early provides the psychological support that is required for rehabilitating the child. Children with stomas resulting from a malignancy usually keep them permanently. Children need to begin learning parts of their care at "potty training" time, which helps them grow into a natural adjustment to the appliances. As children get older, it is vital that they assume complete responsibility for stoma care. The situation is the same as that for diabetic children, who should give themselves their own insulin injections; if the parents do the work and the worrying, the child can use noncompliance or sabotage techniques to manipulate the parents.

Children must be prepared as early as possible to care for their own stoma. If the teaching of ostomy care is included as one of the child's natural developmental tasks, it incurs less frustration and resistance. For example, when children approach two years, or about the time they would normally begin "potty training," they should begin to learn to empty their pouches. To eliminate numerous questions and explanations, children should be encouraged to say "I am going to the potty" rather than "I am going to

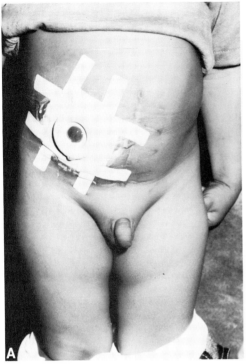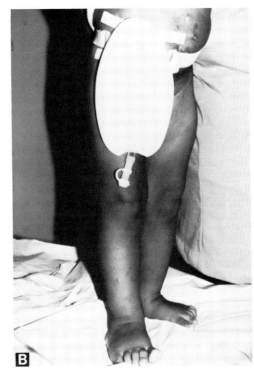

**Figure 11-1.** The parents of this six-year-old boy with an ileal conduit from rhabdomyo-sarcoma of the bladder had alternated getting up twice every night to change his diapers. A two-piece pediatric faceplate (**A**) and pouch (**B**) from United were selected as an appliance for him.

empty my bag." When children begin to be naturally curious in the bathtub and start washing themselves with a sponge or cloth, they can also start washing the area around their stoma. They may need help in removing their pouches—mainly because they may not have the patience to do it gently—but they can begin assisting.

Desires for independence increase in three- and four-year-olds as they learn to dress themselves, and this is an opportune time to promote independence in ostomy care as well. As children develop manual dexterity and learn to use scissors in preschool, they can begin to cut out their adhesives and prepare their pouches. Including play during the teaching makes the sessions less tedious and helps provide relief for small people with short attention spans. Children can begin to practice by cutting pouches and applying them to a doll (Fig. 11-2). Adding stickers and comic characters to the equipment

and pouches is another way of relating ostomy care to the rest of a child's experiences.

By the time children are ready for kindergarten or school, at five, they should be completely able to handle their ostomy care independently. Dependency on parents for stoma care after they have gone to school is far more handicapping to a child than the ostomy itself. Many resources are available to guide the parents, teachers, or nurse of a child with an ostomy (Appendix 11-1). For some, psychological or family counseling may be necessary.

The principles of appliance selection for children are the same as those for adults (see Chapters 2 and 3). The sizes of the plates, pouches, and adhesives are simply smaller (Figs. 11-3 and 11-4). In the early postoperative phase, a skin-barrier wafer may be placed under the appliance. To fit an infant or small child, an adult-size wafer can be cut into fourths and still be large enough to use around the stoma. The

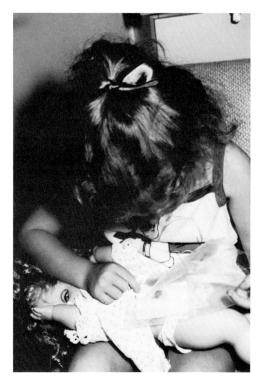

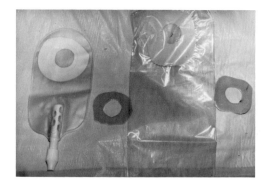

**Figure 11-3.** Skin-barrier wafers cut as small washers and pediatric urinary and colostomy disposable pouches can be applied in the postoperative period.

**Figure 11-2.** A preschooler who had a total pelvic exenteration as a result of sarcoma botyroides practices cutting pouches and applying them to her doll.

appliance and adhesives should be removed gently with warm water, never with harsh soaps, alcohols, or solvents. Because a child's skin is more sensitive to irritation than an adult's, urine or feces that leak onto the skin should be cleaned off promptly and a new appliance applied.

Teaching actual ostomy care to the parents can begin with the first appliance change. Involving the parents early in the care of a child's ostomy helps to reduce their fear of the stoma, and their confidence and calmness are comforting to the child. Children are not as frightened when their mother or father cares for them while the nurse instructs and supervises. After the parents have learned to care for the child, the nurse must continue to give them support and to monitor the condition of the child's stoma and skin—not only while the child is in the hospital but also whenever he or she returns to the clinic.

## URINARY DIVERSIONS

### Ileal Conduits

#### Construction

Since 1950, the ileal conduit has been the most popular form of urinary diversion. The technique of creating an ileal conduit is similar in children and in adults. An isoperistaltic segment of ileum should be used and should be as short as possible to reduce the amount of urine solute reabsorption. As previously stated, the conduit should grow in proportion to the child. The ureters should be spatulated to reduce the likelihood of anastomotic stricture at the ureteroileal anastomosis.

#### Complications

Most of the early complications from ileal conduits are related to errors in surgical technique or judgment (i.e., segment infarction, leaking anastomosis, stomal obstruction, intestinal obstruction, wound dehiscence), but that is not the case with late complications. Over 50 percent of children who undergo ileal conduit urinary diversion have at least one late complication.[11] The most common problems and their incidence (as reported in the literature) are summarized in Table 11-1.

The most frequently encountered late complications are those associated with stomal problems. Neglect and poor hygiene cause most stomal problems, but occasionally stomal com-

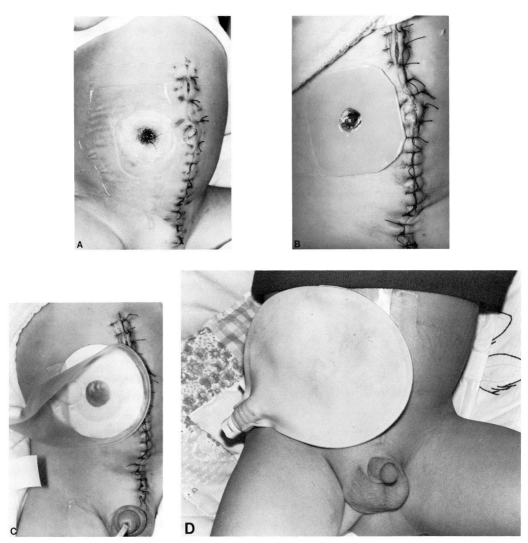

**Figure 11-4.**   **A**, a child with ureterostomies following cystectomy for rhabdomyosarcoma of the prostate. **B**, a skin-barrier wafer applied immediately postsurgically. **C**, a temporary disposable urinary pouch. **D**, the same child fitted with an infant-size reusable urinary appliance.

plications develop in even the most conscientious patient. Most difficulties in the well-constructed urinary stoma are related to alkaline urine causing bleeding, encrustations, and stenosis.[7,14] These difficulties seldom occur in children with poor renal function, possibly because their kidneys produce only dilute urine. In contrast, plaque formation seems to be more frequent in children than in adults, perhaps because of a greater concentrating ability.

*Stomal stenosis.*   The factors leading to stomal stenosis are encrustations and stomatitis, squamous metaplasia, and improper skin segment removal. Some patients, especially blacks, have a tendency to form hypertrophied scars. Sometimes a scarred skin incision merely prevents stomal growth as the child grows, requiring stoma revision.

Two problems may develop with stomal revision. First, the bowel may be too short to

**Table 11-1**
Long-Term Complications of Urinary Diversions in Children

| Ileal Conduits | | Colon Conduits | |
|---|---|---|---|
| Complication | Frequency (%) | Complication | Frequency (%) |
| Stomal problems | 25–42 | Stomal problems | 34–61 |
| Deterioration* | 27–56 | Deterioration* | 36–48 |
| Calculi | 14–30 | Calculi | 14 |
| Ureteroileal stenosis | 7–11 | Ureterocolonic stenosis | 22 |
| Electrolyte imbalance | 1 | Electrolyte imbalance | 1 |
| Pyelonephritis | 12–22 | Ureterocolonic reflux | 51–58 |
| Hypertension | 1 | | |

* Deterioration of anatomical structure visible on intravenous pyelogram.

create the desirable bud stoma, and second, conduit tension may cause angulation of the ureteroileal anastomosis, creating ureteral obstruction. In either situation, a new conduit must be created.

*Stomal encrustation and stomatitis.* Alkaline urine, poor stoma and appliance care, and a high incidence of conduit colonization with a urea-splitting organism, especially a *Proteus* sp., are the major causes of stomal encrustation and stomatitis.

The diameter of the appliance orifice should never exceed the conduit stoma size by more than one-eighth of an inch. The appliance should be removed at least every five days to clean the debris and crystals from the faceplate. Adding vinegar or aspirin to the appliance bag is a good prophylactic measure. High fluid intake to insure dilute urine should be encouraged. Antibiotics should be given as necessary to eradicate urea-splitting bacteria, which increase the alkalinity of the urine.

*Hematuria.* The most common cause of hematuria in children with a urinary diversion is abrasion of the stoma while the child is playing. This is especially common in three- to five-year-old children. Reassurance is usually all that is necessary.

*Loss of renal function.* Perhaps the most discouraging statistic is the clear finding that patients who have a urinary diversion for 10 to 16 years have a 56 percent rate of deterioration in the upper-tract architecture that is visualized on the excretory urogram.[24] For patients who

have the bulk of their life ahead of them, this statistic is devastating.

### Colon Conduits

By 1971, reports from various centers describing large numbers of patients began to document the fate of children with ileal conduits.[4,17,18,21,23–25,27] The occurrence of chronic pyelonephritis and the significant number of late complications associated with ileal conduit diversions prompted surgeons to use the colon to create urinary conduits.[11,29] Paramount in this decision were the technical ease with which an antirefluxing ureteral anastomosis could be created in the colon and the perception that stomal stenosis was less in a colon used for a colostomy. Other expected advantages were lower incidences of ureteral and stomal stenosis, less severe electrolyte disturbances, rapid emptying as a result of mass colonic contraction, and a technically more mobile bowel segment because of a longer mesentery.

Unfortunately, summaries of children who have had colon conduits for at least 10 years seem to show an incidence of complications approximately the same as that in children who have had ileal conduits (Table 11-1).[6,12] Moreover, the entire refluxing mechanism not only seems to fail more than half the time, but also becomes stenotic 22 percent of the time. This ureteroenteral stenosis rate is twice as high as the rate in patients who had a nonrefluxing ureteroileal anastomosis. Finally, it is now clear that patients who have had a ureterosigmoidostomy for over 15 years are at an increased risk of developing a colon carcinoma at the site of the ureterocolic anastomosis.[19,28] Although the most widely accepted theory indicts the admixture of urine and feces, which encourages bacterial activation of endogenously formed *N*-nitrosamine, other mechanisms may be involved that alter local pH arrangements merely by contact of urine with the colon mucosa.[31] Indeed, there is now at least one report of a carcinoma in a colon conduit.[2]

## Summary

Urinary diversions using bowel segments are still the most popular form of diversion in children. Selecting colon over ileum seems to offer no advantage. The child with a urinary diversion needs life-long follow-up, including frequent monitoring of urinary tract anatomy and function.

## Other Forms of Urinary Diversion

For children with cancer who have their pelvic organs removed, supravesical diversion of a permanent nature other than by bowel conduit usually means bilateral cutaneous ureterostomy or unilateral cutaneous ureterostomy and transureteroureterostomy. These types of diversion can be performed only if the ureters are dilated, elongated, and hypertrophied so that they can reach the skin and have a blood supply adequate for survival.[1,5,8,15,16,32]

Occasionally, a temporary diversion is necessary if, for example, the urinary bladder can be spared but has been denervated by the surgical procedure and cannot contract, or if the patient is too ill to undergo an extensive reconstructive procedure (Fig. 11-5).[1,13,16,22] Internal diversions usually have little place in children who have had exenterative surgery, as they require normal rectal function for urinary control. They are usually employed in patients with urinary tract anomalies.

### Cutaneous Ureterostomy and Transureteroureterostomy

The critical requirement for these procedures is the presence of a dilated ureter with a collapsed diameter of at least 1 cm. The advantages of these diversions over a bowel conduit

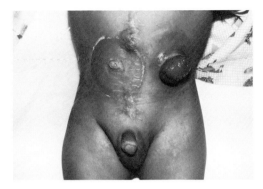

**Figure 11-5.** A child with an obstructing pelvic mass. Cutaneous ureterostomies and a descending loop colostomy were made to relieve the obstruction before chemotherapy was administered.

include decreased operative time, less electrolyte absorption, and possibly a lower incidence of stomal complications.

The stoma should be situated in one or the other iliac fossa. Appliances do not fit well on a midline stoma and interfere more with social functions than do appliances on a laterally placed stoma. When the ureter or ureters are properly spatulated and the wound involves skin flaps rather than a simple skin excision, stomal stenosis can be kept to a minimum.

Stomal problems are usually related to using an undersized ureter or a ureter too short to comfortably reach the skin, thus placing tension on the anastomosis, or to previous radiation damage to the ureter or skin. Acanthosis in these patients is usually attributable to a poorly fitted faceplate or the use of a tight-fitting belt.

### Cutaneous Vesicostomy

Tubeless bladder drainage by a cutaneous vesicostomy, usually using the Blocksom technique, is an easy and fairly trouble-free form of temporary diversion. The bladder is sutured to the skin between the umbilicus and symphysis pubis and the child is kept in diapers. Appliances do not work well with this diversion. It is best used in patients who will later be taught intermittent self-catheterization. The vesicostomy is easily reversible and can be combined with other reconstructive procedures.

*Percutaneous Nephrostomy*

Formal tube nephrostomy has little place in urinary diversion today. Although upper-tract tube diversions are usually a poor choice in children, in the gravely ill child they can be life-saving. In the face of sepsis or azotemia, the surgeon places a catheter percutaneously into the renal pelvis by radiologic, ultrasound, or computed tomographic guidance. Once the acute episode has passed, however, a tubeless form of diversion should be performed, because episodes of bleeding, infection, encrustation, and tube dislodgement are common in this age group.

*Loop Cutaneous Ureterostomy and Cutaneous Pyelostomy*

If a high tubeless diversion is considered, a dilated loop of ureter or the renal pelvis can be brought to the skin quickly. Again, these procedures are rarely indicated in a child who has cancer, but are useful in children with hydronephrosis and hydroureters secondary to congenital anomalies. Appliances cannot easily be placed over these stomas, and flank and upper abdominal diapering are usually necessary. This diversion should be converted, by either performing a more permanent form of diversion or reconstructing the urinary tract, once the episode that precipitated the need for a hastily executed form of diversion has passed.

## ENTERIC DIVERSIONS

Permanent bowel diversions are rarely needed in children, but differ little in construction from those of adults. Most parents place disposable appliance devices over colostomies and ileostomies in the infant. Older children find the temporary appliances to work well for colostomies, but usually need a permanent type of appliance for an ileostomy because of the more liquid nature of the bowel contents.

Temporary colostomies are employed frequently in children with rectal anomalies and are of the loop type. Peristomal hernias are the most common complication of this procedure, which is carried out through a small muscle-splitting incision in the left lower quadrant.

## REHABILITATION

Children with a malignancy that necessitates a bowel diversion, a urinary diversion, or both require continual follow-up care, both emotionally and physically. Every effort should be made for these children to participate in school, recreational activities, and social functions. It is through these that their social education and self-esteem develop.

Parents must become the first line of support. Their attitudes affect their child's perception of himself. If parents are filled with fear, guilt, or embarrassment, children grow to be handicapped with fears, self-consciousness, and low esteem. If, as toddlers, they begin climbing the monkey bars in the park with their friends and their parents are the only ones to rush out in fear and take them down, children will sense that they are different or not strong enough. Their confidence to tackle the next task may be shattered. At first, parents may need assistance in resolving their own fears. Talking to health personnel or to parents of other children with cancer can be very beneficial.

The treatments of malignancies in children carry several potential sequelae. Radiotherapy, chemotherapy, and surgery all may have late effects on growth and development.[9,10] In addition, children who have an ostomy from a pelvic malignancy probably have had their prostate, uterus, or ovaries removed surgically. As these children reach puberty, plans should be made for restorative procedures to alleviate any residual sexual dysfunction.

The physician should discuss genital reconstruction and hormone replacement with parents at the time of the original cancer surgery so that these treatments can be incorporated into the total plan for the child's care. Because genital development and hormone secretions are a natural consequence of puberty, this is the time to incorporate reconstructive treatment into the child's rehabilitation. A girl who has had bilateral oophorectomy should begin taking an oral estrogen at about the age when her mother began to menstruate. She should receive at least a year of hormonal therapy before any surgical reconstruction is attempted. Rarely, a boy has had bilateral orchiectomy for his tumor; if he has, however, he should begin testosterone therapy, which must be administered parenterally, when he is between 13 and 14 years old.

Creating a vagina in a girl and implanting a penile prosthesis in a boy should be delayed until they are at least 15. At that time, the pelvic structures are of a sufficient size to ensure a successful procedure and the patient can share intelligently in the decision to perform the necessary surgery.

No one technique or prosthetic device can be suggested, because each situation is unique. However, if the procedure is delayed past puberty into early adulthood it becomes more difficult emotionally. By then the young man has already experienced the feelings of impotency while his friends are experiencing erections; the young woman has recognized that she has no vagina and has developed feelings of not being ''whole.'' Negative feelings and low self-esteem imprinted during adolescence are difficult to overcome. The health care team and the parents must not overlook sexual rehabilitation—a very important part of the child's total care.

## CONCLUSION

Urinary and bowel diversions, either permanent or temporary, are commonly performed in children with pelvic neoplasms. Proper stomal placement and conduit construction should allow children to perform all normal activities and to conceal their appliances under normal clothing. As early as possible, usually by the age of two years, children should begin to care for their own ostomy, and by the time they are five years old they should be completely in charge.

There does not appear to be an advantage of one type of diversion over another. Stomal stenosis, stomal encrustation, hematuria, and loss of renal function from infection or obstructive uropathy appear to be the major complications of urinary diversions in children.

Emotional support and physical reconstruction of the genitalia are important adjuncts to the total rehabilitation of these patients. Parents must learn to let the children live as normal a life as possible. Sexual rehabilitation at the time of puberty must be part of the efforts of the health team to ensure the patient becomes a well adjusted member of society.

## APPENDIX 11-1

### Resource Material

1. *These Special Children*
   Katherine F. Jeter, Ed.D., E.T.
   Bull Publishing Company
   Box 208
   Palo Alto, CA 94302
   (415) 322-2855

2. *Tommy and His Stoma*
   Ellen Shipes, R.N., M.N., E.T.
   International Urological Services
   P. O. Box 408
   Long Valley, NJ 07853
   (201) 852-8789

3. *The Sneetches and Other Stories*
   Dr. Seuss
   Random House, 1961

4. *A Teenager's Ostomy Guide*
   Bonnie Bollinger, R.N., E.T.
   Hollister, Inc.
   2000 Hollister Drive
   Libertyville, IL 60048

5. *The Physical and Psychosocial Care of Children with Stomas*
   Sharlene J. Hutchinson, R.N., M.S.,
      Ellen A. Shipes, R.N., M.N., E.T.
   Charles C Thomas
   301-327 East Lawrence Ave.
   Springfield, IL

6. *Childhood Malignancy: The Psychosocial Care of the Child and His Family*
   David W. Adams
   Charles C Thomas
   301-327 East Lawrence Avenue
   Springfield, IL
   1980, 200 pp

7. Publications available through United Ostomy Association:
   *All About Jimmy*
   *My Child Has an Ostomy*
   *Colostomies—A Guide*
   *Ileostomies—A Guide*
   *Urinary Ostomies—A Guide*
   Reprints of Articles About Children
      With an Ostomy
   Ostomy Quarterly
   2001 W. Beverly Blvd.
   Los Angeles, CA 90057
   (213) 413-5510

## REFERENCES

1. Burstein JD, Firlit CF: Complications of cutaneous ureterostomy and other cutaneous diversion. Urol Clin North Am 10:433–443, 1983
2. Chiang MS, Minton JP, Clausen K, et al: Carcinoma in a colon conduit urinary diversion. J Urol 127:1185–1187, 1982
3. Cox HT: The cleavage line of skin. Br J Surg 29:231–235, 1941
4. Delgado GE, Muecke EC: Evaluation of 80 cases of ileal conduits in children: Indication, complication and results. J Urol 109:311–314, 1973
5. Eckstein HB, Kapila L: Cutaneous ureterostomy. Br J Urol 42:306–315, 1970
6. Elder DO, Moisey CU, Rees RWM: A long-term follow-up of the colon conduit operation in children. Br J Urol 51:462–465, 1979
7. Filmer RB, Honesty H: Problems with urinary conduit stomas in children. Urol Clin North Am 1:531–547, 1974
8. Flinn RA, King LR, McDonald JH, Clark SS: Cutaneous ureterostomy: An alternative urinary diversion. J Urol 105:358–364, 1971
9. Ghavimi F, Herr H, Jereb B, Exelby PR: Treatment of genitourinary rhabdomyosarcoma in children. J Urol 132:313–319, 1984
10. Hays DM, Raney RB Jr, Lawrence W Jr, et al: Primary chemotherapy in the treatment of children with bladder-prostate tumors in the Intergroup Rhabdomyosarcoma Study (IRS-II). J Pediatr Surg 17:812–820, 1982
11. Hendren WH, Radopoulos D: Complications of ileal loop and colon conduit urinary diversion. Urol Clin North Am 10:451–471, 1983
12. Hill JT, Ransley PG: The colonic conduit: A better method of urinary diversion? Br J Urol 55:629–631, 1983
13. Hurwitz RS, Ehrlich RM: Complications of cutaneous vesicostomy in children. Urol Clin North Am 10:503–508, 1983
14. Jeter K, Bloom S: Management of stomal complications following ileal or colonic conduit operations in children. J Urol 106:425–428, 1971
15. Kogan BA, Gohary MA: Cutaneous ureterostomy as a permanent external urinary diversion in children. J Urol 132:729–731, 1984
16. Leape LL, Holder TM: Temporary tubeless urinary diversions in children. J Pediatr Surg 5:288–303, 1970
17. Malek RS, Burke EC, Deweerd JH: Ileal conduit urinary diversion in children. J Urol 105:892–900, 1971
18. Middleton AW Jr, Hendren WH: Ileal conduits in children at the Massachusetts General Hospital from 1955 to 1970. J Urol 115:591–595, 1976
19. Moorcraft J, DuBoulay CEH, Isaacson P, Atwell JD: Changes in the mucosa of colon conduits with particular reference to the risk of malignant change. Br J Urol 55:185–188, 1983
20. Mosquera G, Devine P: Effect of shape on contraction of abdominal stoma. Invest Urol 12:446–448, 1975
21. Orr JD, Shand JEG, Watters DAK, Kirkland IS: Ileal conduit urinary diversion in children: An assessment of the long-term results. Br J Urol 53:424–427, 1981
22. Perlmutter AD, Patil J: Loop cutaneous ureterostomy in infants and young children: Late results in 32 cases. J Urol 107:655–659, 1972
23. Rabinowitz R, Price SE Jr: Ileal conduit urinary diversion in children. J Urol 114:444–448, 1975
24. Schwartz GR, Jeffs RD: Ileal conduit urinary diversion in children: Computer analysis of follow-up from 2 to 16 years. J Urol 114:285–288, 1975
25. Shapiro SR, Lebowitz R, Colodny AH: Fate of 90 children with ileal conduit urinary diversion a decade later: Analysis of complications, pyelography, renal function and bacteriology. J Urol 114:289–295, 1975
26. Shapiro SR, Peckler MS, Johnston JH: Transureteroureterostomy for urinary diversion in children. Urology 8:35–38, 1976
27. Smith ED: Follow-up study on 150 ileal conduits in children. J Pediatr Surg 7:1–10, 1972
28. Sooriyaarachchi GS, Johnson RO, Carbone PP: Neoplasms of the large bowel following ureterosigmoidostomy. Arch Surg 112:1174–1177, 1977
29. Spence B, Ireland GW, Cass AS: Bacteriuria in intestinal loop urinary diversion in children. J Urol 106:780–781, 1971
30. Stevens PS, Eckstein HB: Ileal conduit urinary diversion in children. Br J Urol 49:379–383, 1977
31. Stewart M, Hill MJ, Pugh RCB, Williams JP: The role of N-nitrosamine in carcinogenesis at the ureteric anastomoses. Br J Urol 53:115–118, 1981
32. Weiss RM, Beland GA, Lattimer JK: Transureteroureterostomy and cutaneous ureterostomy as a form of urinary diversion in children. J Urol 96:155–160, 1966
33. Yu DMC: The physical basis of scar contraction. Plast Reconstr Surg 7:343–351, 1951

Douglas E. Johnson
Dorothy B. Smith

# 12

# Future Considerations

Today, more than 1,500,000 people in the United States and Canada have an ostomy, and estimates are that another 100,000 ostomies will be created during the year, about half of them permanent.[18] Analysis shows that 51 percent of these are colostomies, 36 percent are ileostomies, and 12 percent are urostomies (mainly ileal conduits); less than 2 percent of the patients affected have a combination of two ostomies. For the majority of these patients, the underlying disease necessitating construction of the ostomy is cancer.

Over the past 25 years we have witnessed major advances in the care of patients who have cancer and an ostomy. These advances have resulted largely from improved surgical techniques and better equipment available to care for the stoma. In addition to seeing the quality of life enhanced, we have also watched survival times lengthen markedly for the majority of these patients. Longer survivals have resulted not only from earlier diagnosis and institution of therapy, but also from improved therapies, usually multimodal. Because of these improved therapeutic possibilities, more patients are living for longer periods, prompting physicians to explore ways of eliminating the malignancy while at the same time preserving, or later restoring, urinary and fecal control. In those situations where voluntary continence still cannot be achieved, researchers are attempting to develop methods that will eliminate constant discharge

and, concomitantly, the need for external appliances.

It is not within the scope of this volume to explore all of the innovative procedures currently under investigation. However, as we conclude our discussions of ostomy care for patients who have cancer, we would like to focus attention on the directions in which current research is leading and to comment briefly on the unique problems that the innovative solutions pose to cancer patients.

## URINARY CONTINENCE

### Bladder Substitution

The idea of coupling the contractile power of intestinal segments with the intact sphincter mechanisms of the urethra to reconstruct a new functioning bladder, which appeals to both the forward-looking surgeon and an otherwise reluctant patient, is, surprisingly, not new.[29] The first recorded attempt at such a vesical replacement, using the ileum, was performed by Tizzoni and Poggi in a dog in 1888.[36] However, not until 1951 was the first ureteroileourethroplasty performed in a man.[7] Several investigators[19,26] agreed that the procedure was worth considering for selected patients undergoing radical cystectomy, but other surgeons abandoned the procedure because it compromised good cancer surgery by requiring preservation of a portion of the

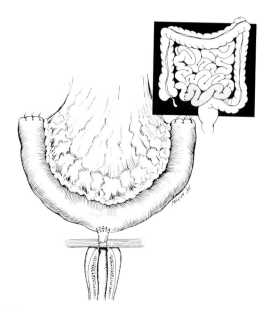

**Figure 12-1.** Ureteroileourethral anastomosis (Camey). A 35- to 40-cm length of terminal ileum is isolated (inset) and the midpoint of its antimesenteric border is anastomosed to the urethral stump. The ureters are implanted, employing an antireflux technique.

prostatic urethra.[3] Furthermore, they found that renal function deteriorated over time.

Recently, the surgical technique has been modified by Camey so that a U-shaped ileocystoplasty is performed, anastomosing the enteric segment to the urethral stump (Fig. 12-1). To date, this procedure has been performed in France in over 400 patients, and its use in this country is becoming more widespread. It allows men to urinate normally through the penis and eliminates the need for an external stoma. However, many patients leak at night unless they are willing to awaken every two or three hours. Leakage can be eliminated by implanting an artificial urinary sphincter.[3]

Other surgeons have constructed a new bladder from an ileocecal segment, a sigmoid colon, or a portion of the stomach and have connected it to the urethral stump, with varying degrees of success.[2,5,8,9,17,23,31]

### Prosthetic Urinary Bladder

The development of a urinary bladder prosthesis has been limited by the availability of structural materials that will not lead to calcifications within the urinary tract. Tsukulidze in Russia pioneered reconstruction with plastic shells and in 1961 reported successfully reconstructing urinary bladders in four patients after total cystectomy.[37] He left a thick shell of polyethene in the pelvis in place of the bladder, implanted the ureters into it, and used a self-retaining urethral catheter to drain the prosthesis. Later, through a second operation, he removed the plastic shell, leaving a fibrous shell that the patient could empty by straining the abdominal muscles and by manual pressure. In a later modification, a polyethene bag that could be drawn out through the urethra was substituted for the plastic shell, thus eliminating the need for the second operation.

Recently, Kline and Eckstein[20] at the University of Miami have constructed an artificial implantable bladder of polyether urethane and Dacron mesh. The bladder consists of a flexible diaphragm that is attached to a stiff, cup-like base and that fills and empties by natural gravitational and peristaltic forces. The ureters are anastomosed to nipples extending from the base of the prosthesis. Normal ureteral peristalsis fills the prosthesis, and voiding is regulated by a manually controlled valve incorporated into its foundation. It is predicted that a prototype of this bladder prosthesis may be ready for clinical trials within five years.

### Continent Cutaneous Urostomy

Problems in achieving total urinary continence encountered with a variety of enteroure-thral anastomoses have prompted other investigators to explore the possibility of constructing a continent intraabdominal reservoir that could be emptied by periodic urethral catheterization, thus obviating an external urinary appliance. Gilchrist and associates[12,13,33] have reported satisfactory use of the ileocecal segment (Fig. 12-2), but other physicians have not been able to achieve consistent continence in their patients, in spite of modifying the technique in a variety of ways.[1,4,14,25]

Encouraged by his results with the continent ileostomy reservoir, Kock[22] was prompted to adapt the reservoir for cutaneous urinary diversion (Fig. 12-3). His initial experience with 12 patients convinced him that urinary diversion via a continent ileal reservoir offered the patient a quality of life much superior to that achieved with conventional urinary diversion procedures. This early success gave impetus to others[11,24,32] to use the procedure, and as a result the technique is gaining favor as an alternative to the more frequently performed ileal conduit.

## BOWEL CONTINENCE

### Colostomy Continence

Numerous attempts have been made over the years to control the bowel movements of ostomates by means of prosthetic devices. An analysis of the various approaches[35] shows that they fall into one of four categories: (1) external devices, (2) surgical techniques alone, (3) surgical techniques plus passive implanted devices, and (4) surgical techniques plus active implanted devices. Although it is not within the scope of this book to discuss these techniques in detail, we do want to point out the wide range and creative variety of the procedures employed. They include a single inflatable cuff (cuff end of a tracheostomy tube) inserted into the stoma;[35] an implantable hydraulic sphincter prosthesis around the bowel;[34] an inflatable plastic balloon placed in the subcutaneous tissue around the stoma;[15] a samarium-cobalt magnetic ring encased in either methyl methacrylate or titanium placed around the bowel and a separate cap containing a magnetic core (magnetic stoma cap);[10] a silicone ring implanted within the peritoneal cavity to serve as a buttress for a silicone balloon plug (Fig. 12-4);[28] and a surgically created seromuscular sleeve that is freely transplanted around the external bowel wall several centimeters proximal to the site of the stoma.[30] When Schmidt[30] reviewed the experience with over 500 patients in whom the seromuscular sleeve was employed, he reported that approximately 80 percent did not require an external appliance and "nearly all viewed their postoperative situation as markedly improved." Corman,[6] although quick to note that experience has been limited and the follow-up period short, believes that Plager's continent colostomy plug holds promise, especially since there are no absolute restrictions on the type of patient who is a candidate for the procedure and side effects appear nonexistent. The other devices and procedures have generally proved disappointing because their complication rates are high and they

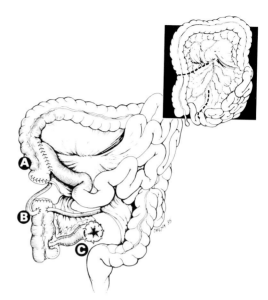

**Figure 12-2.** Ileocecal bladder (Gilchrist). The proposed incisions in the mesentery are indicated by the dotted lines in the inset. The completed procedure shows the ileocolostomy *(A)*, the ureters implanted into the proximal ascending colon, which has been oversewn *(B)*, and the terminal ileum brought out at the stoma *(C)*.

have failed to achieve continence for many patients.

### Ileostomy Continence

Because of the problems associated with a conventional ileostomy (skin irritation, difficulties managing appliances, and psychological disabilities), Kock[21] devised a "low pressure" continent ileal reservoir for patients who have had a proctocolectomy. The principles of the procedure have already been illustrated in Figure 12-3. The operation is technically complex and is fraught with many complications, including failure to achieve continence, which have required reoperation in 6 percent to 25 percent of the patients who have tried it. However, experience can significantly reduce the high complication rate, and the procedure is offering a markedly improved quality of life to many patients.

An attractive alternative for selected pa-

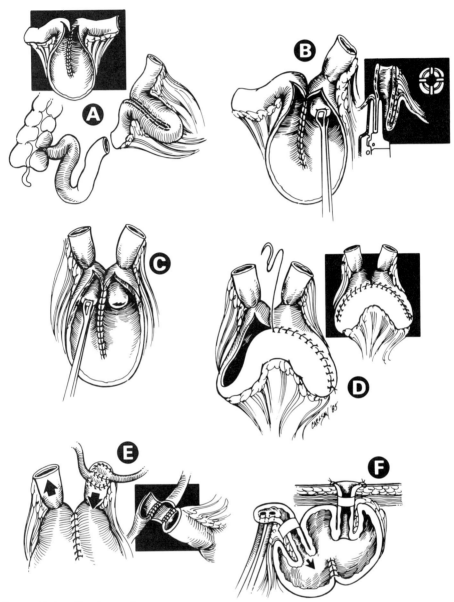

**Figure 12-3.** Continent ileal reservoir (Kock). **A**, 60 to 70 cm of ileum is isolated approximately 50 cm from the ileocecal valve. The legs of the U are united at the antimesenteric border and then opened along the suture line (inset). **B** and **C**, the afferent and efferent segments are intussuscepted and the nipple valves fixed with the stapling instrument (inset). **D**, the reservoir is closed. **E**, the ureters are implanted into the inlet segment. **F**, the completed reservoir in situ.

tients who require a proctocolectomy is the construction of an ileal reservoir and ileoanal anastomosis (Fig. 12-5).[27,38] The procedure, modeled after the successful Kock reservoir, utilizes an ileal pouch to eliminate propulsion activity and to act as a storage receptacle. This procedure also carries with it a high morbidity, but operative deaths have been few. In spite of its problems, most patients who have accepted the procedure have preferred life with the ileal-anal anastomosis to life with an ileostomy.[16]

## SPECIAL CONSIDERATIONS FOR PATIENTS WITH CANCER

Although the techniques that preserve or restore urinary and bowel continence are mark-edly improving the quality of life for some patients who, heretofore, would have required conventional ostomy surgery, these procedures are often contraindicated, unfortunately, in pa-tients who have malignant disease. Cancer pa-tients frequently require multimodal therapy (surgery, chemotherapy, and radiotherapy) to eradicate their disease. They can ill afford oper-ative procedures that prevent their receiving a part of their coordinated therapy at the appro-priate time. This is especially true of patients undergoing radical cystectomy for invasive blad-der cancer, where the use of postoperative ad-juvant chemotherapy appears to significantly lengthen survival. The Kock pouch may appear to be an ideal solution for patients whose blad-der is removed, but the increased morbidity associated with the procedure and the high reoperative rate required to achieve urinary con-tinence restrict its use to patients who are un-likely to need adjuvant chemotherapy.

The presence of artificially constructed res-ervoirs or implantable prostheses poses major concerns about the postsurgical treatment of cancer patients. Those who undergo radical cystectomy or colectomy usually have advanced disease and either need to receive chemotherapy adjuvantly or require it later for metastatic dis-ease. Newly constructed reservoirs (Kock uri-nary pouch, Camey procedure, etc.) do not have the inherent mechanisms for controlling infec-tion that are normally present in the intact bladder. Futhermore, since the isolated bowel acts as a reservoir rather than as a conduit, residual urine is always present. The result is

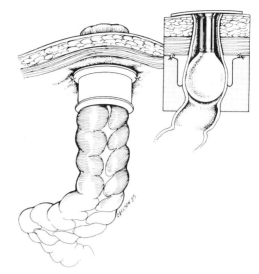

**Figure 12-4.** Continent colostomy plug (Pla-ger). A silicone ring with a flange is implanted in the peritoneal cavity and sewn onto the undersurface of the abdominal wall. The colon passes through the ring and a stoma is created in the usual manner. Inset: the plug in position.

stasis and almost universal pyuria. Pyuria itself is not a major concern to an asymptomatic person, but to an immunosuppressed and myelosuppressed cancer patient who is receiv-ing chemotherapy, it can pose a major threat. Similarly, even though implantable prostheses are purposely made of inert material, they can serve as a nidus for infection in a debilitated cancer patient.

The Camey procedure, which preserves uri-nary control, is contraindicated in another set of patients—those whose bladder malignancy is multifocal, encroaches on the bladder neck, or involves the prostatic urethra and ducts. Pa-tients with bladder cancer at these sites are at high risk for developing urethral recurrences, and therefore urethrectomy is usually indicated at the time of radical cystectomy. Similarly, an ileal reservoir combined with an ileoanal anas-tomosis is seldom applicable in patients with colorectal carcinoma, because these patients usually require a total colectomy to prevent local recurrences. Even if the risk of anal recur-rence could be eliminated, the increased morbid-ity of the procedure would preclude the use of

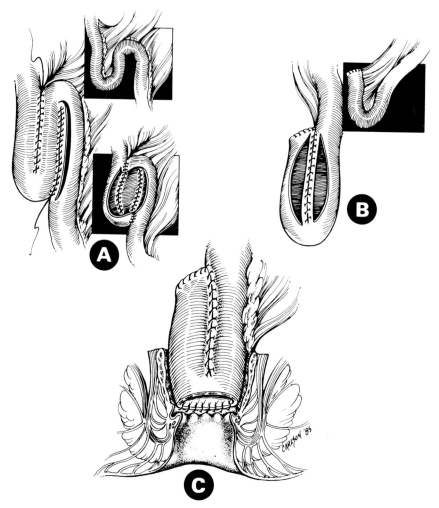

**Figure 12-5.** Ileal reservoirs and an ileoanal anastomosis. **A**, an S-type ileal reservoir. **B**, a J-type reservoir. **C**, the completed ileoanal anastomosis, showing the newly constructed pouch brought down endorectally to the anal canal, preserving the anal sphincters.

early postoperative adjuvant therapy. In addition, the presence of the small bowel in the pelvic region limits the amount of postoperative radiotherapy that can be delivered safely.

## CONCLUSIONS

Although some of the recent developments in surgical techniques and in construction of inert artificial prosthetic devices have succeeded in controlling urinary and fecal flow, their application for patients with cancer appears to be severely restricted. While we remain concerned about the quality of life, we must keep the eradication of the malignancy as our first concern; quality of life cannot exist without life! For the present, the morbidity and risks of these procedures, much greater than those of conventional therapy, would place the majority of cancer patients in jeopardy by adversely affecting their therapy.

Standard ostomy surgery remains the simplest, safest, and most expedient method today for treating patients who have malignant disease. Consequently, good stomal care provides for our patients the best quality of life attainable at the present time.

## REFERENCES

1. Ashken MA: An appliance-free ileocecal urinary diversion: Preliminary communication. Br J Urol 46:631–638, 1974
2. Baker R, Carrol P, Hayes D: Sigmoid segment for bladder substitute after total or subtotal cystectomy. J Urol 90:289–295, 1963
3. Barry JM, Petre TM, Hodges CV: Ureteroileourethrostomy: A 16-year followup. J Urol 115:29–31, 1976
4. Benchekroun A: Continent caecal bladder. Br J Urol 54:505–506, 1982
5. Charghi A, Charbonneau J, Gauthier GE: Colocystoplasty for bladder enlargement and bladder substitution: A study of late results in 31 cases. J Urol 97:849–856, 1967
6. Corman ML: Colon and Rectal Surgery. Philadelphia, J. B. Lippincott, 1984, p 652
7. Couvelaire R: Le réservoir iléal de substitution après la cystectomie totale chez l'homme. J Urol (Paris) 57:408–417, 1951
8. Cukier J: La cystectomie totale avec cellulectomie du petit bassin (note technique). J Urol Nephrol (Paris) 73:231, 1967
9. Diokno AC, Sonda LP, MacGregor RJ: Long-term followup of the artificial urinary sphincter. J Urol 131:1084–1086, 1984
10. Feustil H, Hennig G: Continent Kolostomi durch Magnet Verschluss. Dtsch Med Wochenschr 100:1063–1064, 1975
11. Gerber A: The Kock continent ileal reservoir: An alternative to the conventional urostomy. J Enterostom Ther 12(1):15–17, 1985
12. Gilchrist RK, Merricks JW: Construction of a substitute bladder and urethra. Surg Clin North Am 36:1131–1143, 1956
13. Gilchrist RK, Merricks JW, Hamlin HH, Rieger IT: Construction of a substitute bladder and urethra. Surg Gynecol Obstet 90:752–760, 1950
14. Harper JGM, Berman MH, Hertzberg AD, et al: Observations on the use of the cecum as a substitute urinary bladder. J Urol 71:600–602, 1954
15. Heibum M, Cordoba A: An artificial sphincter: A preliminary report. Dis Colon Rectum 21:562–566, 1978
16. Heppell J, Kelly KA, Phillips SF, et al: Physiologic aspects of continence after colectomy, mucosal proctectomy, and endorectal ileo-anal anastomosis. Ann Surg 195:435–443, 1982
17. Hradec E: Bladder substitution: Indications and results in 114 operations. J Urol 94:406–417, 1965
18. Hurny C, Holland J: Psychosocial sequelae of ostomies in cancer patients. CA 35:170–183, 1985
19. Kirkegaard P, Lyndrup J, Walter S, Poulsen PE: Long-term results after uretero-ileo-urethrostomy. Br J Urol 54:226–229, 1982
20. Kline J: Implantable prosthetic bladder works without external power. Urology Times 13:31, 1985
21. Kock NG: Intra-abdominal "reservoir" in patients with permanent ileostomy. Preliminary observations on a procedure resulting in fecal "continence" in five ileostomy patients. Arch Surg 99:223–231, 1969
22. Kock NG, Nilson AE, Nilsson LO, et al: Urinary diversion via a continent ileal reservoir: Clinical results in 12 patients. J Urol 128:244–250, 1982
23. Lilien OM, Camey M: 25-year experience with replacement of the human bladder (Camey procedure). J Urol 132:886–891, 1984
24. Madigan MR: The continent ileostomy and the isolated ileal bladder. Ann R Coll Surg Engl 58:62–69, 1976
25. Mansson W: The continent caecal reservoir for urine. Scand J Urol Nephrol 85(Suppl):1–137, 1985
26. Mellinger GT, Suder GL: Ileal reservoir (ureteroileourethral anastomosis). Method of urinary diversion. JAMA 167:2183–2186, 1958
27. Parks AG, Nicholls RJ: Proctocolectomy without ileostomy for ulcerative colitis. Br Med J 2:85–88, 1978
28. Prager E: The continent colostomy. Dis Colon Rectum 27:235–237, 1984
29. Sarma KP: Tumors of the Urinary Bladder. London, Butterworth, 1969, p 343
30. Schmidt E: The continent colostomy. World J Surg 6:805–809, 1982
31. Sinaiko ES: Artificial bladder from a gastric pouch. Surg Gynecol Obstet 111:155–162, 1960
32. Skinner DG, Boyd SD, Lieskovsky G: Clinical experience with the Kock continent ileal reservoir for urinary diversion. J Urol 132:1101–1107, 1984
33. Sullivan H, Gilchrist RK, Merricks JW: Ileocecal substitute bladder: Long-term followup. J Urol 109:43–45, 1973
34. Szincz G: A new implantable sphincter prosthesis for artificial anus. Int J Artif Organs 3:358–362, 1980
35. Tenney JB, Graney MJ: The quest for continence: A morphologic survey of approaches to a continent colostomy. Dis Colon Rectum 21:522–533, 1978
36. Tizzoni G, Poggi A: Die Wiederherstellung der Harnblase. Zentralb Chir 15:921–924, 1888
37. Tsulukidze AP: On the treatment of patients with bladder tumors. Urol (Mosk) 28:43–49, 1963
38. Utsunomiya J, Iwama T, Imajo M, et al: Total colectomy, mucosal proctectomy and ileoanal anastomosis. Dis Colon Rectum 23:459–466, 1980

# Index